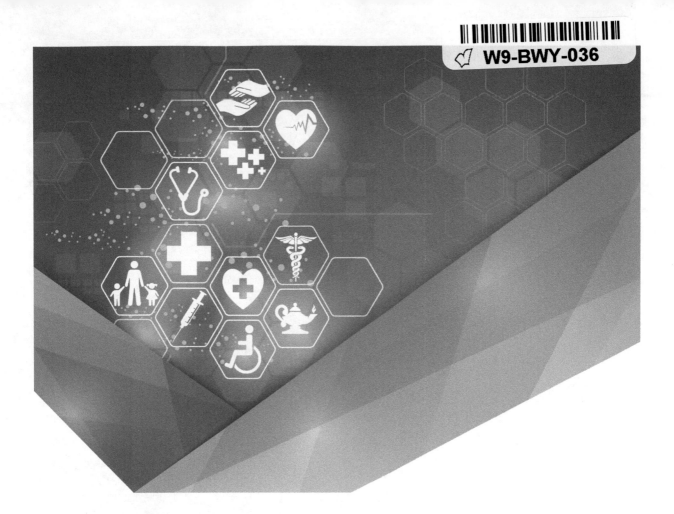

ETHICAL
COMPETENCY
IN NURSING &
ALLIED HEALTH

GERALDINE HIDER & DON HOEPFER

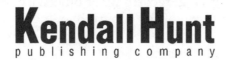

Kendall Hunt
publishing company

Cover design created by Scott Gore

Kendall Hunt
publishing company

www.kendallhunt.com
Send all inquiries to:
4050 Westmark Drive
Dubuque, IA 52004-1840

DEDICATION

For Rebekah Pringle and Ian Pringle. It wasn't so much where we needed to be but it was the pathway with many turns of how we arrived. My endearing gratitude for you and your unconditional love was worth the journey.

For Josh Goss and Kaycee Goss. Philosophy operates in words, yet its discoveries move deeper. There is profound and renewing discovery in my children of choice.

In memory of Julie Hoepfer. She gave more than she endured. This book is possible because of her.

TABLE OF CONTENTS

INTRODUCTION

Ethics is for you. It's an active process that involves all of us. It is more than acknowledging your feelings and beliefs. Ethics brings you to consider different perspectives, analyze a situation, and think critically about what you should do and who you should be. This book will help you with the ethics portion of a test you will take for licensure. Most of all, this book is designed to be a bridge that links you from deskside to bedside; a source for your professional career.

Assessments are commonly performed in the everyday practice of nurses and allied health professionals. You do physical assessments when you first encounter a patient. In the same way when you face a moral issue, you can do an ethical assessment. Competency in ethics sharpens your ability to discern nuanced ways to view the situation and the perspectives of various people involved, and to think critically about appropriate ways to address that situation.

The book is offered in two parts. Chapters 1 through 3 develop an Ethical Assessment Model. The authors don't intend to make *ethics* easy. The intention is to present ethical decision-making so that it can be done with competency and some degree of confidence.

Chapter 1 draws out a correlation between ethics and safety. The book opens with an exploration into *first do no harm* as a foundational ethical issue. Often, the perception of harm results in a reaction of negative moral judgment.

Our moral reactions, however, are not always reliable guides to ethical behavior. Moral feelings and beliefs can be biased and short-sighted. Critical thinking and other skills can help to place our feelings in context and aid in the development of better understanding, which can lead to better behavior and better outcomes. Chapter 2 examines these skills as part of ethical competency.

The skills of ethical competency benefit from taking on the perspectives of different levels of assessment: administrative, strategic, and interpersonal. These levels are explored in Chapter 3 through the use of normative ethical theory and features of everyday practice. The chapter closes with an Ethical Assessment Model to help guide the process of analyzing a moral situation through these different levels.

The second part of the book, Chapters 4 through 11, provides application for the model. There is an association between ethical competency and integrity. The skills of ethical thinking and action combine to help cultivate wholeness in you as a professional and as an individual. Professional oaths and codes of ethics, along with a multileveled approach to ethical thinking, can provide guidance toward integrity. This is the focus of Chapter 4.

The first application of health care is toward the patient, toward the one who suffers. In being exposed to risk, a patient looks for traits in those who provide care. A patient looks for professionals who are trustworthy, who will speak the truth with compassion, who will act with fidelity, and who will respect the patient's needs for privacy and confidentiality. These traits are components of giving voice to a patient's needs. This is advocacy, the focus of Chapter 5.

Cultivating integrity implies accepting responsibility for your behavior. There are policies and protocols that you are responsible to follow. Deeper than these is the way you value the safety of your patients, your coworkers, and yourself. This is part of developing a culture of safety, the topic of Chapter 6.

Stress and uncertainty are a given in health care, and in life. Stress and burnout can manifest in various forms of moral dejection. Chapter 7 explores the manner in which empathy presents exposure to risk of moral dejection and provides the key to managing this risk through compassion.

Professional integrity impacts upon the way in which you participate with coworkers. There are virtues of communication that contribute to good outcomes and cultivate respect. Chapter 8 explores the ethics of collaboration, including the importance of preventing horizontal and vertical violence.

Chapter 9 examines integrity under extreme duress, when all that is normal is disrupted. The processes of large-scale disaster and disease for an individual bear parallels to each other.

Advocacy can be directed toward a specific patient and for human society as a whole. Chapter 10 examines social justice, exploring the way in which professional obligations toward a single person can impact concerns for fairness, equality, diversity, and the avoidance of stigma.

Health and health care are of interest to us. We value health so much that we tend to take it for granted when we have it. Typically, we only reflect on health when it is absent or when it has just been restored. Bioethics is an effort to bring more reflection to health, for the purpose of better elevation of humanity. The contributions of nursing and allied health professionals to this reflection are explored in Chapter 11.

The purpose of the book is to help bring the process of ethics to your professional and personal life. The Ethical Assessment Model is a means to help gain perspective, clarity and a better way of seeing a moral situation. Ethics is open-ended. Ethics is that style of thinking that is employed when there is something of moral value at stake in the midst of a situation saturated in ambiguity. There is room to discuss, explore, and wonder. These are skills that are part of ethical competency. The Ethical Assessment Model, and this book as whole, is not intended to present ethical decision-making as a way to always provide a clear path to a single right answer. The situations that challenge us morally do so because they present complicated circumstances that can be approached with different viewpoints. Ethical competency provides a way to navigate this complexity and not be paralyzed into inaction.

The academic style of this book is to engage readers in a process of exploring ideas. Each chapter begins with a list of objectives that describe areas of exploration. Chapters do not have the objective to provide final answers to moral questions, but to provide the skills that can be used in the practice of addressing moral situations.

Exercises and Case Studies are included at the ends of chapters and interspersed throughout the chapters. While some might have clear answers, all are designed to inspire further thought, conversation, and exploration. As you engage these, concentrate less on arriving at a right answer and more on the process of exploration. Use case studies as an opportunity to build perspective and gain practice in the use of the Ethical Assessment Model. Use the exercises as ways to explore and refine your own moral beliefs.

If specific dates are given, then an example or exercise is factual and drawn from history or from news accounts. All other examples, exercises and case studies are hypothetical. All names are derived from the use of random name generators.

ACKNOWLEDGEMENTS

Special thanks to Scott Gore for our cover design. (Do you see the butterfly?) We are pleased to have a friend and colleague with his talent and kindness. For more about this artist, please visit Gore Studios, https://facebook.com/gorestudios/.

Thanks to Marissa Morris, Kara Perella and Steve Moore. Your ongoing support and encouragement is uplifting.

To Kerri Milliken: *thanks, and thanks, and ever thanks.* Because of you, in many ways, future generations will have much to read. Thanks also to others who helped with copy editing: Sarah Star, Christopher Kurfess, Jeanne Hoecker, Padraig Davitt, and Dianna Parks.

Thank you to everyone at Kendall Hunt for their support and guidance. Thanks to Angela Lampe for first seeing worth in the project. Special thanks go to Michelle Bahr and to Reveilee Lanning for their responsiveness, advice, and frequent conference calls. Thanks, too, for the warm welcome when we visited Kendall Hunt's main office.

Over the course of writing this book, we talked about our project with many people, including Olive and Esther. Your encouragement and enthusiasm were sustaining and affirming. For all those we encountered: Thank you. We met as strangers and left as friends.

To all of our students and attendees at our conference presentations: You were part of ongoing efforts to explore ideas. There is no better way to learn than to teach. Thank you. It is always a joy to work with you.

To Tim Johnson and other patients: Some were recipients of our care. Some we sat beside in clinic waiting rooms and in support group meetings. Your suffering has not gone unnoticed. What you endured matters because it happened to you. What you endured matters because it will have a healing impact on others.

Special thanks to Jennifer, who played a bigger part in this than she will ever know.

ABOUT THE AUTHORS

Working night shifts as a nurse, Geraldine Hider encountered stillness. The daytime bustle of a hospital floor subsided; it was just her patients and her. Over a period of nine years, Don Hoepfer's wife encountered darkness. She endured two cancer diagnoses, multiple surgeries and chemotherapeutic regimens, several clinical trials, and hospice care. In stillness and darkness, the authors were with people who suffered; who gave voice to their fear, distress, pain, anger and anxiety.

This book represents the combined perspective and research of two authors who observed the profound importance of a nuanced ethical approach in attending to patients in their vulnerability. Illness can be a profoundly philosophical experience. The authors work to combine philosophical insight with clinical practicality that recognizes the importance of melding compassion with attention to principles, procedures, and outcome analysis.

Geraldine Hider is a registered nurse. She has worked in clinical research, critical care, operating room, peri-operative care, pediatrics, procedure room nursing, floor nursing, and palliative and hospice care. She has advanced degrees in Disaster Medicine and in Management.

Don Hoepfer is a professor of philosophy at a community college. His experience as a caregiver and his philosophical research into illness led to the development of a philosophy and cancer course. He has an advanced degree in Philosophy and is pursuing a degree in Bioethics.

FIRST, DO NO HARM

OBJECTIVES

After completing this chapter, you will be able to . . .

1. Explain harm as a foundational principle of ethics in health care.

2. Identify and apply the four principles of biomedical ethics: autonomy, nonmaleficence, beneficence, and justice.

3. Discern the difference between ethical thinking and moral reactions.

4. Demonstrate practical understanding of the interplay among your moral feelings, your professional duties, and your ethical analysis.

KEY TERMS

- Autonomy
- Beneficence
- Empathy
- Ethical competency
- Ethics
- Executive control
- Harm
- Justice
- Moral conflict
- Morality
- Moralize
- Nonmaleficence
- Normative
- Rationalize
- Suffering

> ### *Respect the inherent dignity and worth of every person*
>
> A health information management professional shall:
>
> - Treat each person in a respectful fashion, being mindful of individual differences and cultural and ethnic diversity.
> - Promote the value of self-determination for each individual.
> - Value all kinds and classes of people equitably, deal effectively with all races, cultures, disabilities, ages, and genders.
> - Ensure all voices are listened to and respected (AHIMA, (2011).

INTRODUCTION

First, do no harm.

Despite the common assumption, this statement doesn't come from the Hippocratic Oath. Something like it can be found in Hippocrates' *Epidemics,* written around 400 BCE. Here, Hippocrates states that *a physician should have two main goals in mind when treating disease:* be of benefit or, at least, do no **harm** (Jones, 1981, p. 165).

Harm is damage or offense experienced by a person.

This sentiment is not unique to Hippocrates. We can see it in many philosophical writings, in many religions, and in many professional codes of conduct. There's a commonsense appeal to this idea. *At the very least, try to not cause harm.*

The idea that we should avoid causing harm seems obvious. Even so, it's not entirely clear as a moral directive. Does this mean that you should avoid causing harm at all possible costs? Does it mean that you should focus on doing good and should only worry about not causing harm if you face circumstances in which you can't produce much good? If you have to make a choice between protecting yourself from harm and preventing harm to someone else, what should you do?

Ethics does not suppose that there are always easy answers to our questions about what we ought to do and the kind of people we ought to be. Ethics does suppose that it is worthwhile to explore these questions. When should we sacrifice some good in order to avoid causing harm? Under what circumstances is it justifiable to allow some harm as we attempt to create some benefit? As mentioned in the introduction to this book, ethics confronts ambiguity in our lives—those times when we don't know what to do and we feel something of value is at stake. We refine this idea a little more here. We turn to ethics when we face ambiguity and sense that the choice we make can bring some benefit or at least avoid some harm.

EXERCISE

Make a list of some of your moral convictions. You can write them as "I believe that . . ." Once you have your list, look over what you have written. How many of these statements are consistent with: "Be of benefit or, at least, do no harm"?

Facing a situation of significance, we take notice when we see someone being harmed (Figure 1.1).

For the most part, we experience an intuitive, negative reaction when we witness someone experience harm. **Empathy** is a common ability in us to recognize suffering in others and to feel a measure of pain ourselves in response. The pain the observer feels mirrors, but does not exactly duplicate, the pain felt by the other person. The observer recognizes that the other person is in pain and the pain felt by the observer amounts to an emotional connection. The emotional content and the interpersonal connection may produce some motivation on the part of the observer to reach out and offer aid to the person in pain (Schaich Borg, 2016). While we typically associate empathy with a response to pain, we can also recognize that we have the capacity to react positively to the alleviation of **suffering** and to rescuing someone from possible harm.

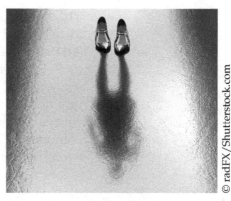

Figure 1.1 You can walk in someone's shoes, but you still use your own feet

© radFX/Shutterstock.com

These positive and negative reactions are significant. Our negative responses to the perception of harm show that we take an interest in avoiding suffering. Actions that are wrong cause, or fail to prevent, someone from being harmed. Actions that are good somehow prevent or alleviate harm. Typically, we prefer actions that offer some benefit with small risk of known harms than actions that promise great benefit with risk of significant or unknown harms.

Our positive responses indicate that we also take an interest in experiences beyond harm and suffering. In other words, there is something we look for in our lives that we are best able to experience without harm and suffering getting in the way. We can call this positive interest an interest in well-being.

Empathy is an experience that follows the observation of pain in another. This experience is characterized by a feeling of pain on the part of the observer that mirrors the pain felt by the other person.

Suffering is a quality of personal experience characterized by pain, distress, or other negative perceptions.

EXERCISE

Suffering has just been equated with harm. Do you see any important difference between suffering and being harmed? Can you think of any examples in which someone suffered but has not been harmed?

There are some who believe that avoiding harm is the main unifying idea behind ethics (Goodwin, 2017; Royzman, Goodwin, & Leeman, 2011). Such a view holds that *all* moral questions ultimately come down to a consideration of harm. If we are to promote that idea that all ethics involved thinking about harm, then we need to be very broad in our definition of *harm*. Obviously, causing someone physical damage counts as harm. Do you also cause harm to someone you neglect? If someone's rights are violated, are they harmed? Can you be harmed even if you never know it?

EXERCISE

A patient is not consented for a procedure. The patient never knew that consent should have been obtained. We will say that the patient's rights to autonomy have been violated. However, the patient, ignorant of other options or the requirements for consent, is satisfied with the procedure and does not believe that any harm has been done. Has the patient been harmed? Imagine that the patient later learns that there has been a violation and becomes upset. Has the patient been harmed? If so, when did the harm occur? Was it when the patient *felt* upset? Would there be any harm if the patient learned about the violation and didn't mind that it occurred?

Another way to look at the notion that avoiding harm is the unifying idea of ethics is to consider all people—indeed, all living beings—as suffering in some way. We carry our physical hurts with us. We suffer from emotional pain and stress. We face problems, worries, and frustrations. All is not well with us in every respect. Perhaps, it is our most basic moral calling to address all of this suffering as best as we are able.

Consider a passage from Śāntideva's *The Way of the Bodhisattva*:

> *For all those ailing in the world,*
> *Until their every sickness has been healed,*
> *May I myself become for them*
> *The doctor, nurse, the medicine itself. Source:* Śāntideva (2008), p. 48.

Śāntideva asks us to think of everyone in the world as a patient. In nursing and allied health, we are presently faced with patients. Śāntideva offers illness (harm) as a way to see each person as having moral value. Look to each person as your patient. In crafting this image, Śāntideva is expressing harm as a unifying idea of ethics. We can look at all our moral actions as efforts to reduce suffering in the world.

Even if the global reach of Śāntideva's vow doesn't speak to you, as a health-care professional, you can connect with the vow on a practical level.

EXERCISE

Compare Śāntideva's vow with Hippocrates' advice to be of benefit or at least do no harm. What similarities and differences do you see between them? Use this discussion to think about what kind of moral direction would be helpful to you.

Adding one more voice to the *first do no harm* chorus: "The very first requirement in a hospital is that it should do the sick no harm." This is from Florence Nightingale, in her book *Notes on Hospitals* (Nightingale, 1863, p.1).

Nightingale's career and writings identified ethical conflicts in the existing standards of care for patients. Hospitals during her time lacked policy and procedures for patient care. There were no regulatory agencies overseeing health-care standards, and protocols were nonexistent for nursing staff. She asserted herself as an advocate for patients within hospitals whose methods were unsafe and unsanitary. She identified the moral importance of patient dignity and safety. The spirit of her work to establish the value of taking all care to avoid causing harm to patients can be found in today's policies and procedures.

Nightingale's first writings to nurses were more in the way of guidelines. She believed that morality came from within the person and ethics addressed the wholeness for providing care.

Whether or not *all* ethics is oriented toward harm is debatable. The writing and advocacy of Florence Nightingale, the guidance of Hippocrates, and the imagery of Śāntideva all point to harm as a foundational ethical concern in health care. We readily acknowledge health as good and illness and injury as sources of suffering (harm). The various healthcare professions are dedicated to helping people maintain health and to address suffering by promoting healing and reducing pain and suffering.

EXERCISE

Disease is clearly a source of suffering. Disease processes harm the body and cause physical, emotional, and social distress. Do you believe that addressing a patient's disease is inherently moral? Do you believe that disease is always a moral challenge?

The emergence of a field of dedicated ethical attention to health care—bioethics—maintains a focus on harm. The last chapter of this book will provide a brief historical sketch of harm in medicine and the development of bioethics. For now, we will turn our attention to a central portion of one of the most cited works in the field, the four principles in Beauchamp and Childress' classic text, *Principles of Biomedical Ethics* (Beauchamp & Childress, 2016).

FOUR PRINCIPLES

Beauchamp and Childress' principles are highly influential in bioethics. In a field as diverse as ethics, the influence of these principles is quite remarkable. These principles are a common source of appeal in the field of bioethics and for decision-making in the clinical setting. (Gillon, 2003). These principles are at the heart of the *Occupational Therapy Code of Ethics* (AOTA, 2015). The principles are also highlighted in the American Nurses Association's *Code of Ethics for Nurses with Interpretive Statements* (American Nurses Association, 2015). The principles are explicitly covered in many publications relating to health care.[1] The concepts expressed in these principles will be readily identified in far more publications and in many discussions about bioethics. In sum: professionals in nursing and allied health will need to know these principles.

Each of the four principles—autonomy, nonmaleficence, beneficence, and justice—will be articulated with respect to harm as a foundational ethical concept.

AUTONOMY

Autonomy literally means *self-rule*. As a moral principle, it calls upon us to respect the rights of individuals to think for themselves and determine the course of their lives. In health care, respect for autonomy means informing patients and acknowledging that they have the final say about their own treatment

> **Autonomy** is a principle of respect for an individual's right and capacity to make choices that help to determine the course of that individual's life.

Principle 3 of the AOTA Principles and Standards of Conduct: Autonomy

Occupational therapy personnel shall respect the right of the individual to self-determination, privacy, confidentiality, and consent.

Autonomy is rooted in the regard we have for individuals. To be an individual means that your life is your own. You should have the authority to decide for yourself where you will go, what you will do, and who you will be. No one should be able to force you into a major purchase, into a career, or into a major life decision.

Treatment decisions, of course, can count as major life decisions. Respect for autonomy means acknowledging patients' own authority over what is done to their bodies. Autonomy further means that patients should have some authority over their own illness. Autonomous patients make the decisions that they deem to be best for them. They might decide against a recommended treatment. They might opt out of treatment altogether.

The necessity of obtaining consent from patients has not always been an accepted standard in health care. It has been believed that patients need confidence in a healer. Having one who asks permission before treatment might yield unwarranted anxiety in a patient. It has also been argued that patients simply don't have the expertise that doctors possess (Murray, 1990). Who is in better position to determine whether one treatment option or the other is the better choice?

Concerns about the lack of medical expertise of patients drive an important part of autonomy: informed consent. Consent refers to the patient's choice. Patients should be asked if they agree to procedures before

---

[1] A Google Scholar search turned up over 23,000 citations. https://scholar.google.com/scholar?hl=en&as_sdt=0%2C39&q=principles+of+biomedical+ethics+beauchamp+and+childress&oq=%22principles+of+biomedical+ethics

they are performed on them. Health-care professionals have the added responsibility to make sure that patients have some reasonable basis from which to make this choice. They need to be informed about the procedure, about alternatives, about risks, and about a realistic expectation of benefits. Patients will still not have the expertise of the doctor. However, in wondering which of the two—patient or doctor—is in the best position to make a treatment decision, the answer is generally taken to be, *Both of them, Together.*

Respecting autonomy means that patients should have the authority to make their own decisions. You can expect that you will interact with patients who make decisions with which you disagree. You might believe that a patient could receive a better health outcome if only a different choice were made. In such circumstances, you might wonder if autonomy means allowing the patient to come to harm.

We now face a question of the nature of harm. Imagine that a patient is declining treatment that would assuredly bring about a good health outcome. By refusing this treatment, the patient is going to suffer. As you view it, this is needless suffering. As you wonder about this, someone reminds you of the principle of autonomy: "How much harm would this patient suffer if a treatment decision was imposed and the person had no choice?" The principle of autonomy is built on the ethical notion of rights. Under this notion, it is argued that there are essential ways in which humans ought to be respected. If that respect is violated, there is harm to the person at a very fundamental level. This might not manifest as physical harm but the offense is there just the same. More, when human rights are violated, all of humanity is in some way harmed by the offense. What we do to each other affects us all. To paraphrase one of the most important writings of twentieth-century philosophy: *A violation of human rights anywhere is a threat to humanity everywhere.*[2]

EXERCISE

Are there physical manifestations when human rights are violated? Think about ways in which people can suffer if they are denied authority over their own lives. Can some of these consequences present as physical suffering?

---

[2] The original is "Injustice anywhere is a threat to justice everywhere." It is from Dr. Martin Luther King, Jr.'s "Letter from Birmingham Jail". King, M. L, & Carson, C. (1998). *The autobiography of Martin Luther King, Jr.* New York: Intellectual Properties Management in association with Warner Books. Print.

EXERCISE

Are there physical manifestations when human rights are violated? Think about ways in which people can suffer if they are denied authority over their own lives. Can some of these consequences present as physical suffering?

NONMALEFICENCE

Thus, we come back to the beginning of the book. *First do no harm* is an essential statement of **nonmaleficence**. The term *maleficent* refers to acts that inherently cause harm. Realistically, we cannot expect to act so as to cause no harm whatsoever. The point is to do one's best to act thoughtfully and avoid causing needless harm.

> **Nonmaleficence** is a principle that affirms our responsibility to avoid causing needless harm to persons.

We raise nonmaleficence as something of an obvious point in morality. Don't harm people. Don't leave them worse than you found them. Even though it seems an obvious point, it is a point that needs raising. Imagine that a patient of yours has died. You are packing up that patient's belongings. You didn't know this patient, but you hold a pair of shoes and a few articles of clothing. A person wore these. How did this person leave this world? How do you hope this person left this world?

Florence Nightingale placed nonmaleficence as the core of nursing ethics. Nightingale's work brought to light practices that raised risks of harm to patients. Hippocrates stressed the importance of not harming patients. His admonition was directed to physicians who engaged practices that caused harm. Nightingale and Hippocrates weren't in the habit of merely stating the obvious. They raised concerns about maleficent acts because they recognized that they were occurring.

Principle 2 of the AOTA Principles and Standards of Conduct: Nonmaleficence

Occupational therapy personnel shall refrain from actions that cause harm.

In some contexts, maleficence is associated with evil. Certainly, we can see that it is a horrible thing to intentionally cause someone harm for no reason other than to cause harm. This is a hard line that we can draw. Don't do this.

But nonmaleficence doesn't only call us away from such wickedness. The principle is especially calling upon us to be mindful of the fact that our actions can have effects beyond what we intend. Florence Nightingale wasn't accusing hospital personnel of consciously seeking to cause people to suffer. She pointed out that many practices within a hospital caused suffering. She drew attention to these issues with the expectation that reasonable people would agree with her insight and that changes would be made.

The principle of nonmaleficence has its power in calling upon us to think hard about how we act. We can easily focus on the good we intend to do for each other. This is fine—it is, in fact, the next principle—but we are not always aware of the full reach and consequence of these actions. Nonmaleficence is a cautionary principle at its heart. When we promote this principle, we do not do so because we anticipate evil. We do so because we know that we need to cultivate a broader scope of awareness. Our actions can have risks that we might not initially see.

EXERCISE

How much conflict is fueled by moral controversy? How do the different sides of these conflicts view each other? Do these people anticipate evil from each other?

BENEFICENCE

From the Latin word *bene*, this principle calls upon us to act for the good of others. This is the spirit of Nightingale's work, Śāntideva's vow, and of Hippocrates' first main goal in treating disease: be of benefit.

Beneficence | **Beneficence** is the complement of nonmaleficence. Where nonmaleficence is the duty to take all due caution to ensure that you are not a source of harm to the patient, beneficence is the duty to do good for patients by bringing them benefit or by keeping them harm.

Beneficence
is a principle
that affirms the
importance of doing
good.

As with nonmaleficence, beneficence is not merely a direct matter of intending to do good. In health care, beneficence directs us to promote good health outcomes. Think of all the ways in which this can be done. In alleviating pain or stopping a disease process, we do good by bringing an end to a cause of suffering. In the case of treating trauma, we do someone good by rescuing them from immediate danger. Immunization programs do good by preventing harm from occurring. We can do good by providing continuing care for those who suffer from chronic illness or disability. We can do good for disadvantaged populations—and for humanity as a whole—when we advocate for justice and respect for rights (Beauchamp & Childress, 2016, p. 204).[3]

There is a connection between beneficence and harm. The connection itself has two main layers. Beneficence is a "desire to do good." In this sense, giving pain medication promptly to spare a patient from suffering is beneficent. This pertains to Śāntideva's call to embody the doctor, the nurse, and the medicine in an effort to manage the patient's suffering. Beneficence further entails taking care to remove sources of harm from the patient and to protect the patient from further sources of harm.

Principle 1 of the AOTA Principles and Standards of Conduct: Beneficence

Occupational therapy personnel shall demonstrate a concern for the well-being and safety of the recipients of their services.

JUSTICE

Inequalities in access to health care and to public health services place individuals and populations at risk. Lack of sanitation creates the risk of disease. Areas prone to malaria can suffer economically as large portions of the workforce lose time with illness. Income inequality correlates with increased rates of poor health (Fiscella, Franks, Gold, &, Clancy, 2000) and mortality (Kawachi, Kennedy, Lochner, & Prothrow-Stith, 1997).

Principles aim to provide guidance for us all equally. **Justice** is the principle that affirms the need to promote equality as we make available the services and benefits that health care can provide.

In a few of his dialogues, notably in the *Meno* and in the *Republic*, Plato tackles what must have been a popular adage of the time: Justice is helping your friends and harming your enemies. Showing little patience for this idea, Plato works to show that, while helping your friends is a lovely thing to do, harming anyone is not a suitable intention for any person of justice. Among the lines of reasoning that Plato employs is the observation that harming enemies has consequences beyond the harm done to the enemy. Your enemy might strike back at you in retaliation. If the enemy has been so damaged that retaliation is not possible, then this enemy is going to present a drain on other resources. In a way, damage done to an enemy is damage done to all.

Justice is a principle requiring fair and equitable distribution of resources, including access to health-care services.

---

[3] Beauchamp, Tom L., and James F. Childress. *Principles of Biomedical Ethics*. 2016. Print. Page p. 204.

It is better, if possible, to try to enlist an enemy as a friend. Doing so, you are able to derive the greater benefit—you have turned a threat into an advantage.

Principle 4 of the AOTA Principles and Standards of Conduct

Occupational therapy personnel shall promote fairness and objectivity in the provision of occupational therapy services.

Following Plato, we can easily say that purposefully causing inequities is not consistent with justice. The harm to the disadvantaged populations will be bad enough, but the whole society will suffer from economic inefficiency, public health risks, and deleterious effects.

The more insidious problem will be inequities that arise systemically. These inequities involve a confluence of factors such as geography, poverty, language barriers, educational opportunities, transportation availability, assumptions about gender and gender roles, access to healthy food and other goods that are essential to a healthful lifestyle, and other goods. For instance, people who live in *food deserts* live in urban areas in which there are few places to purchase wholesome, nutritious foods. The cost of the food and the means to travel to these stores makes purchasing nutritious food prohibitive. In food deserts, people rely on food obtained from convenience stores and gas stations. These foods are relatively affordable but also high in fat and processed sugars. Children who grow up in such an environment may face problems with obesity and malnutrition stemming from a poor-quality diet. Faced with better opportunities, these children might have been given a better diet, but those opportunities are not available in the areas where these children live. While not intentional, these systemic issues can develop as a product of discrimination, stigmatization, or other practices that fail to respect equal worth of persons. A social system that we think is just can contain elements of oppression that establish inequalities and prevent affected populations from overcoming those elements (Frye, 1983).

The principle of justice promotes efforts to bring equality and opportunity to all without disparity based on discrimination, neglect, or disadvantage. Justice is a goal of working to balance social goods and opportunities, with the idea that this works toward the benefit of every individual as well as toward society as a whole. In the interest of justice, we should reach out to those who are disadvantaged so as to connect them with opportunities to participate in a society of individuals with comparable equality. Because inequities can be hidden or insidious, the exercise of the principle of justice needs to be on something of a watchdog role.

ĖXERCISE

Research the Tuskegee Syphilis Study. Explain the problem that this study posed from each of the four principles: Autonomy, Nonmaleficence, Beneficence, and Justice.

ETHICS AND MORALITY

In this book, we will use harm as the cornerstone of our exploration into ethics. We are here to do what we can to benefit those who are suffering and to avoid causing them harm.

The place to start our exploration is to clarify some concepts. We have all heard and used terms like *morality* and *ethics*. How often do we think about what they actually mean?

Morality refers to the beliefs you hold about values as they apply to human behavior. We express these values in terms of dichotomies such as good/bad, right/wrong, and moral/immoral. Morality is one way of seeing value in your world. It's what you believe and how you feel. It includes the abilities to form, and act on, certain beliefs. These beliefs pertain to right and wrong, values and priorities, and your images of who you are and who you ought to be.

Moral beliefs can be viewed in two ways that we often confuse. Morality can be *descriptive*, pertaining to the beliefs that a person has about appropriate behavior. Morality can also be **normative** and used in judgment to assert that people ought to accept and practice a certain belief about appropriate behavior. Here, you hold an expectation that people ought to accept and act on a moral belief.

Normative moral beliefs can be the products of our intuitions, feelings, and unchallenged tenets. For this reason, judgments from moral beliefs are prone to be reactionary, superficial, and biased. From these beliefs, we can engage in **moralizing**—pushing one's own moral beliefs as the only proper way of seeing things. The mark of moralizing is a self-righteous attitude and a relatively closed mind.

Ethics is an activity of critical thinking in which we examine beliefs about morality and the processes by which we come to have our moral beliefs. Ethical thinking involves gathering information, considering different perspectives, carefully evaluating different viewpoints, and testing hypotheses. Ethical thinking makes use

Morality consists of beliefs you hold about values as they apply to human behavior.

Normative is a term that describes the promotion or determination of a standard, or the evaluation of a standard. Normative ethics consists of efforts to help us determine how we should act.

Moralize to moralize is to take on an air of authority in professing your opinions about morality. It is to act as if others should regard your moral standards as the standards they ought to accept.

Ethics is an activity of critical thinking in which we examine beliefs about morality and the processes by which we come to have our moral beliefs.

of several decision-making tools. Included among these decision-making tools are principles (such as autonomy, beneficence, non-maleficence, and justice), assessment of possible outcomes, and attributes (such as care and compassion) that facilitate interpersonal connection.

Ethics can be normative as well. However, ethics, should be an open-minded approach. Ethical assessments will often take a stand, but we should still be open to reconsideration as new perspectives and new information are presented. This is because ethics is the concerted activity of questioning what we ought to believe. Ethics looks to possibilities and options. Beliefs set through ethical thinking should be beliefs that are thought out and that can be adjusted, strengthened, explained and defended.

The essential difference between morality and ethics is the difference between having beliefs and thinking carefully about what your beliefs ought to be. It is the difference between acting on the basis of your feelings and instincts and pausing to determine how you ought to act.

Specifically, for our purposes, we will further think of morality and ethics in terms of harm. Actions that are moral are those that bring benefit and avoid causing harm. Actions that are immoral cause harm while failing to bring benefit. Ethics involves the careful and deliberative act of examining a situation in which harm is at stake in an effort to arrive at a course of action that seems best suited to bringing about benefit and avoiding unnecessary harm. Judgment from ethical assessment is like a judge's verdict—considered, deliberative, and offered from expanded perspective.

Ethical thinking is a skill. The effort to develop its abilities includes rational deliberation about theoretical matters, charitably entertaining different perspectives and putting them in their best light, applying logical critique to ideas and arguments, listening and discussing with others, reviewing your actions, introspection over your values and beliefs. These efforts—and more—constitute ethics.

Moral beliefs can vary across cultures. They can vary among individuals. They can be influenced and shaped by religion, social economic status, group affinity and history, personal history, and many other factors.

Moral beliefs can change over time. People sometimes think there is strength in standing by one's beliefs no matter what, but this might not be a realistic expectation. Your moral beliefs have changed over time. This happens as you learn new things, encounter new situations, pursue your education, mature, and take on new perspectives. Change can be good, when you make an informed, thoughtful choice. Ethics is a practice that prepares you to change your beliefs about morality when necessary, and it can help you to otherwise enhance your understanding. Ethics is an ongoing endeavor.

MORAL INTUITIONS

Neuroscience is revealing much about processes involved in perceiving moral issues and making moral decisions. Research shows that there is no single moral center in the brain. Rather, morality is processed in multiple areas of the brain. These centers also process such phenomena as emotion, motivation, cognition, perspective-taking, and awareness of others (de Oliviera-Souza, Zahn, & Moll, 2017).

Moral intuition is a fast response to a perception that is experienced as having moral significance. We are sensitive to perceptions of harm. When we also perceive someone's intent behind the harm, our moral attention activates. Within the brain, the posterior superior temporal sulcus (pSTS), amygdala, and ventromedial prefrontal cortex (vmPFC) activate successively within 400 milliseconds. In that short period of time, your experience carries information about intent and intervention, associates an emotional affect to the situation, produces some motivation toward the situation, and generates some cognitive interpretation of the event and people involved (Decety, & Cacioppo, 2012). As a comparison, an eye blink lasts up to 400 milliseconds. When you witness a moral event, you form an initial moral perception in the same span of time as a blink of your eye. This is fast enough that you experience your moral reaction as intuitive. This is so fast that it arrives with a perception of certainty because you have not entertained doubts or engaged in any deliberation. The emotional content, which precedes cognitive content, lends itself to your possible response, "I feel . . ." (Decety, & Cacioppo, 2012).

The experience of *intent* is a perception that the agent who caused harm knew that harm would result from that agent's action and was motivated in some way to cause that harm. Notice the way in which we commonly regard intentional harm as worse than harm that is produced accidentally.

Intending to cause harm is not always immoral. Part of our judgment depends on whether harm was the primary motivator or a secondary effect behind a different, more noble, intention. Giving an injection with a hypodermic needle may cause pain, but the act can readily be morally justified. In this case, the intention is not to cause harm. The presence of harm attracts attention. We are less likely to judge an act as wrong if we see that the primary intent behind the action was not to cause that harm.

Regardless of perceptions of intent, our attention is captured when we see one agent intervene and forcibly alter the movement of another. Pushing someone off their path is an example. Another example is stopping someone in their motion or compelling someone to move who otherwise appears to wish to stay still. When the intervention causes harm, we process the situation as having moral content (Nagel & Waldman, 2012; Waldmann, Wiegmann, & Nagel, 2017). When we also perceive intent to intervene and cause harm, we react negatively toward the agent who causes the harm (Schaich Borg, Hynes, Van Horn, Grafton, & Sinnott-Armstrong, 2006).

In August, 2017, a BBC video became a sensation on YouTube. The video showed a female pedestrian narrowly escape traumatic injury when a jogger passing the other way shoved her to the side. She fell so that her head extended into a traffic lane, right in front of an oncoming bus. The bus driver swerved just enough to avoid striking the fallen woman (BBC News, 2017). The sight of the jogger pushing the woman elicits a shocked reaction in many who view the video. It is easy to feel immediate moral judgment directed against this jogger.

EXERCISE

For a straight-forward example of intervention, consider this scenario: You are walking down a hallway and reach an intersection. Someone else reaches the intersection at the same time and bumps into you, pushing you off your path and into a wall. Do you imagine that you would initially be upset and ready to blame the other person for pushing you? What would you need to know in order to decide whether or not you should actually blame the other person?

Experienced as a feeling or intuition this response is immediate and fresh. It arises with ready appeal. Your attitude and affect are already set. Your mind is made up. You don't have to spend much energy on this apart from the emotional energy that is part of your reaction. Moreover, since this reaction comes intuitively—that is, without the expense of a conscious thought process that entertains options—it arises with an air of certainty (Kahneman & Frederick, 2005).

No other choices are presented. You react *this* way and no other. The belief arises immediately, establishing a powerful connection to the moral issue at hand. Moreover, the belief is emotionally charged. This is what you believe. This is what you feel. Very often, these feelings are very strong. The reaction will either be *Yes! This is the right thing to do* or *No! This is wrong!!* This reaction comes with emotional force.

There is a lesson in the way that you come to have moral beliefs. For the most part, your moral beliefs serve you well. Most of the time, your moral beliefs help to shape your experience and guide your behavior. This happens without much need for thought. Forming moral intuitions is a nonconscious brain event. In many instances, we feel these intuitions so strongly that we arrive at reasons to justify our intuitions.

Often, we stick with our moral beliefs because we *make* those beliefs make sense to us. We can invest so much in these intuitions and the reasons we offer to justify them that we often see no reason to change our minds—no matter what other arguments and perspectives are offered.

Research shows that people tend to reinforce inclinations with choices. Such choices can amount to **rationalizations** (Schwitzgebel & Ellis, 2017). Ethics involves more than making you feel better about your initial reaction to a moral event. Ethics entails full exercise of **executive control**—the capacities to investigate your reactions, to deliberate about them, and to arrive at a position that might be very different. Think about why you might see a need to change your beliefs. Moral intuition doesn't operate on a full view. It operates on what attracts your attention right away—a *perception* of harm along with force and intent that produces motivation and cognitive description. The motivation and cognitive can be described as shallow because you don't see the issue from all possible angles from this immediate perception.

But you often encounter situations where you don't know what to do. You also find situations in which your initial reactions don't accurately assess the circumstances. Your moral beliefs, in other words, sometimes aren't enough, no matter how much you try to make them make sense. Sometimes, your moral beliefs can actually be inaccurate or incomplete and lead to action that cannot be supported ethically. A reactionary moral stance does not take full consideration of the situation and, therefore, could fail to adequately respond to critical circumstances. Errors can follow. These errors could lead to further moral complications. Errors can lead to hard feelings among other people involved in the situation. Errors in assessing circumstances can contribute to poor health outcomes for patients. Errors in moral judgment can have legal consequences, or professional consequences such as loss of licensure.

To be clear, none of this is meant to say that your moral feelings are wrong. As we will see, there is a place for your feelings and intuitive beliefs in assessing a moral issue. The point to grasp is that your feelings are a starting point. Ethics is a process, and your feelings are an initial step in that process.

ETHICS AND THINKING ABOUT MORAL INTUITIONS

You have a lot more to offer than just your moral intuition. A moral intuition will be based only on a quick assessment of what you observe. This view can be flawed. It will almost certainly be incomplete. A moral intuition comes with conviction, but the strength of your conviction is no guarantee of accuracy or understanding. Even though you have a belief that *feels right*, you could still be mistaken in that belief.

Rationalize to rationalize is to attempt to justify one's behavior by offering reasons that sound plausible but really don't hold up to logical scrutiny.

Executive control consists of consciously directed cognitive processes that modulate other processes in order to pursue certain goals.

Moral intuition happens without choice. This does not mean, however, that you cannot exercise choice once you have your immediate reaction to a moral event. *Choice* engages processes of executive control. Choice is the power to reinforce the inclinations that are produced in moral intuition or to modify or overrule them.

Often, we limit our sense of morality to what we feel. While our feelings are obviously an essential part of our moral lives, these feelings can create problems. You will encounter conflicts between your beliefs and those of others. There might be conflicts between your feelings and procedures you are expected to follow.

Here's the good news: You are not stuck with your intuitions. For all that your moral intuitions arise without choice and bear the force of certainty, they can be modulated.

We know that moral judgments can be influenced by external factors. The way that moral problems are posed can bias the way that people interpret them. Feelings of discomfort or disgust can make people harsher in their moral judgments. Your moral judgments are not simply facts about the world. They are also statements about what you feel at the time. If you influence someone's feelings and perception, you can influence that person's moral intuitions.

There are many ways to modulate the moral reactions of your brain. Among these modulations is conscious deliberation. You can think rationally. You can gather information. Gain perspective. You can refine your beliefs and feelings. We know that moral intuitions are subject to modification by executive functions in the brain. You are not fated to the moral feelings that you have. You can think about them and change your mind as warranted. You can also develop a richer idea of why you feel the way you do.

HEART/HAND/HEAD MODEL

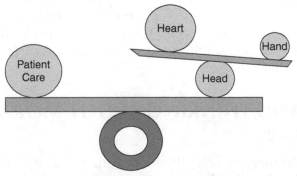

Figure 1.2 Heart/Hand/Head Model

The Heart/Hand/Head model (Figure 1.2) points to some of the complexity about us as we face acting ethically. Human beings interface with the world on many levels, in many different roles, and with different faculties. The *heart, hand, head* imagery points to three faculties that we use as we engage our moral lives. The reference to anatomy is metaphoric, of course. We have moral reactions to events we witness and to people that we care about. This is represented with the *heart*. We have tasks and expectations that are set for us by our jobs, by law, and by the expectations of other people in our lives. There are routines that guide our actions. In many ways, we act from a practical, procedural standpoint. This is represented by the *hand*. We also have the faculty to be creative, to be intellectual, to think critically. This is represented by the *head*.

The *heart* represents that activity within us in which we naturally and immediately place value. Here are our felt values, tastes, attachments, desires and dreams. In most circumstances, it is the heart that speaks first. Think to the times when you have an immediate value-laden reaction to something that happened. You can think that your actions are moral here, because you instinctively act according to your beliefs.

The *hand* represents that activity within us in which we opt to set aside our own decision-making and follow the rules, regulations or duties given by someone else. The hand is able to push down the heart's force and pick up the mantle of duty. You can think that your actions are moral here because you are following the rules that you have been taught.

The *head* represents that activity within us in which we charitably entertain competing ideas, weigh them carefully and decide on a course of action. This involves critical thinking. This is where you work to attain balance.

When we act with the heart, we react intuitively and emotionally to the situations we face. When we act with the hand, we closely follow what we have been told or advised to do. When we act with the head, we think about what we do. We conceive of options. We inquire. We research. We reason. *We consult the heart and the hand*. This is where ethics happens.

This process seeks balance. Rely too much on moral reactions (heart) or rote action (hand) and mistakes can be made. Harm can result. The work of ethics is to maintain awareness of what you feel and what you are required to do. There are ways to engage this process so as to maintain your awareness and to think carefully and thoughtfully in order to conduct yourself as best you can in your moral world.

Your moral world also needs you to help establish balance. The heart/hand/head model acknowledges that your moral actions do not just affect you. Doing ethics is not only in your own interest, it has impact on others. Your balance can help maintain or restore balance for others. Your ethical actions, in other words, can make a profound difference for your patient.

Think about how you seek balance now. Where do you find it in your life? Who helps you to find it? Think about your vision for yourself as a professional. How can your actions help someone else to find balance?

At the beginning of this chapter, it was argued that harm is fundamental to ethics in health care. While harm is the main concern of ethics in health care, *conflict* often precipitates the occasion for doing ethics in health care. Much of what we do is happily consistent with what ethical inquiry will recommend. On an ordinary basis, we find heart and hand in agreement. The head is often not occupied with ethical judgments about what occupies heart and hand. That is, our moral intuitions and feelings usually fit with the procedures we are expected to follow. For the most part, what we do meets with no controversy and no confusion. It is when we perceive conflict that we acutely find the need to think about ethics.

Moral conflict A moral conflict is the perception of an inconsistency between a moral value of your own and either the values of someone else or a situation in which you cannot successfully act to promote your moral value.

Moral conflict takes many forms. In the experience of a moral event, there may be conflict between what you witness and your intuitive sense that harm should not be intended nor forced upon someone. In such a case, your ethical assessment might be consistent with your moral intuition. The more troubling forms of conflict arise when your moral intuitions are somehow confounded. You might find conflict between your moral intuition and the procedures you are expected to follow. You might find conflict between your moral intuition and the intuitions of someone else. Some conflicts will take the form of an ethical dilemma in which you have two or more options from which to choose, yet none of these options enables you to bring about all the moral good you wish to produce. No matter what you choose, you leave behind some option that might have produced a certain good that your chosen option won't produce.

See that there are many aspects to ethics. There is the need to attend to regulations and duties set by outside sources. Above all, there is the need to bring your feelings and these external duties into an overall process in which you think carefully about the circumstances you face. Here, you identify what you should do and who you should be.

In his *Phaedrus*, Plato describes the soul as having three parts—desire, conscience, and rationality. To illustrate the proper relationship between these, he uses the imagery of a chariot drawn by two horses. One horse is noble and obedient. The other is full of fire. As a team, they are a mismatch. The wild horse always wants to fly, especially when it sees something it wants. The other horse waits for commands from the charioteer, and so the wild horse is trying by itself to drag the chariot and its teammate along. The quieter horse tries to hold its ground when the wild horse takes off, and it wins when the wild horse is exhausted. This pairing doesn't work. The vital element here is the charioteer who will have to work carefully, persistently, and diligently to try to reign in the wild horse. This will be hard work, but it is necessary in order to bring harmony to the team. Only in this way can the chariot reach its destination.

The wild horse represents desire—for us, the heart. The quiet horse represents conscience—that which holds us back and gives us time to set aside our feelings for the commands of others. For us, this is the hand. The charioteer is the head. Notice that this illustration shows that the head does not dismiss the heart or the hand. Both have essential roles to play in thinking ethically. You must pay attention to your feelings and to regulations and protocols. But you must also think. *Above all*, you must think. Otherwise, you are always following, at the mercy of one horse or another.

This is to suggest that **ethical competency** can do more than help you figure out the right thing to do. There will be hard choices to make. There will be no-win situations and ethical dilemmas in which it is hard to identify one action that is absolutely right. We cannot always arrive at a story book ending. Thinking ethically not only helps us to make decisions; it also helps us to take stock of hard feelings, exhaustion, guilt, and remorse that can follow a particularly difficult situation. Ethical competency can help to restore of a sense of balance.

> **Ethical competency** is proficiency in cultivating and exercising the skills of inquiring into issues of human morality.

REFERENCES

AHIMA. (2011). *AHIMA code of ethics*. Chicago, IL: American Health Information Management Association. Retrieved from http://bok.ahima.org/doc?oid=105098#.Wt55DtPwau5

American Nurses Association. (2015). *Code of ethics for nurses with interpretive statements*.

AOTA. (2015). Occupational therapy code of ethics (2015). *American Journal of Occupational Therapy, 69,* 6913410030p1–6913410030p8.

BBC News. (August 8, 2017). *Jogger 'pushed' woman in front of bus—BBC News*. YouTube. Retrieved from https://www.youtube.com/watch?v=OuuHrVhykD4

Beauchamp, T. L., & Childress, J. F. (2013). *Principles of biomedical ethics* (7th ed.). New York: Oxford University Press.

de Oliviera-Souza, R., Zahn, R., & Moll, J. (2017). Neural correlates of human morality: An overview. In J. Decety, & T. Wheatley (Eds.). *The moral brain: A multidisciplinary perspective.* (pp. 183–195). Cambridge, MA: MIT Press.

Decety, J., & Cacioppo, S. (2012). The speed of morality: A high-density electrical neuroimaging study. *Journal of Neurophysiology*, 108(11), 3068–3072.

Fiscella, K., Franks, P., Gold, M. R., & Clancy, C. M. (2000). Inequality in quality: addressing socioeconomic, racial, and ethnic disparities in health care. *JAMA 283*(19), 2579–2584.

Taylor, V., Whittier, N., & Rupp, L. (Eds.) (2012). *Feminist frontiers*. New York: McGraw-Hill. (Reprinted from Frye, M. (1983). Oppression. In *The politics of reality: essays in feminist theory*.)

Gillon, R. (2003). Ethics needs principles—four can encompass the rest—and respect for autonomy should be "first among equals". *Journal of Medical Ethics*, 29(5), 307–312.

Goodwin, G. P. (2017). Is morality unified, and does this matter for moral reasoning? In J.-F. Bonnefon & B. Trémolière (Eds.). *Moral inferences* (pp. 9–36). New York: Routledge.

Hippocrates. Jones, W. H. S., Trans. (1923). *Hippocrates volume 1*. In Loeb Classical Library, No. 147 Cambridge, MA: Harvard University Press.

Kahneman, D., & Frederick, S. (2005). A model of heuristic judgment. In K. J. Holyoak & R. G. Morrison (Eds.). *The Cambridge handbook of thinking and reasoning* (pp. 267–293). New York, NY: Cambridge University Press.

Kawachi, I., Kennedy, B. P., Lochner, K., & Prothrow-Stith, D. (1997). Social capital, income inequality, and mortality." *American Journal of Public Health, 87*(9), 1491–1498.

Murray, P. M. (1990). The history of informed consent. *The Iowa Orthopaedic Journal, 10*, 104.

Nagel, J., & Waldman, M. (2012). Force dynamics as a basis for moral intuitions. *Proceedings of the Cognitive Science Society, 34*, 785–790. Retrieved from http://escholarship.org/uc/item/1r88v2x0

Nightingale, F. (1863). *Notes on hospitals*. Longman, Green, Longman, Roberts, and Green.

Royzman, E. B., Goodwin, G. P., & Leeman, R. F. (2011). When sentimental rules collide: "Norms with feelings" in the dilemmatic context. *Cognition 121*(1), 101–114.

Śāntideva. (2008). *The way of the Bodhisattva* (p. 48). Boston, MA: Shambhala Publication.

Schaich Borg, J. (2016). The influence of rodent models of empathy on human models of harm prevention. In S. M. Liao (Eds.). *Moral brains: The neuroscience of morality* (pp. 246–277). New York: Oxford University Press.

Schaich Borg, J., Hynes, C., Van Horn, J., Grafton, S., & Sinnott-Armstrong, W. (2006). Consequences, action, and intention as factors in moral judgments: An fMRI investigation. *Journal of Cognitive Neuroscience*, 18(5), 803–817.

Schwitzgebel, E., & Ellis, J. (2017). Rationalization in moral and philosophical thought. In J.-F. Bonnefon & B. Trémolière (Eds.). *Moral inferences* (pp. 170–190). New York: Routledge.

Waldmann, M. R., Wiegmann, A., & Nagel, J. (2017). Causal models mediate moral inferences. In J.-F. Bonnefon & B. Trémolière (Eds.). *Moral inferences* (pp. 45–63). Hove: Psychology Press.

CHAPTER 2

ETHICAL COMPETENCY

OBJECTIVES

After completing this chapter, you will be able to . . .

1. Identify the skills of ethical competency and contemplate how they may be implemented into one's practical life.

2. Implement the processes of critical thinking when doing an ethical assessment.

3. Demonstrate comprehension of what it means to be a moral agent and the goal of ethical competency in moral agency.

4. Identify and review different justifications for ethical reasoning and the development of ethical competency.

5. Explain each of the four vital intentions and apply them in ethical reasoning.

KEY TERMS

- Building perspective
- Critical thinking
- Gathering facts
- Humility

- Moral agent
- Normative ethics
- Reciprocity

The cytotechnologist understands that the responsibility for the welfare of the patient supersedes responsibility to all others. The cytotechnologist acting in a professional manner shall: exercise ethical judgment in decision-making processes, accept the responsibility for the consequences of these decisions, and be able to acknowledge personal error. Abide by the rules and regulations of the laboratory or institution (ASCT, 2006).

INTRODUCTION

There are cognitive and affective skills involved in ethical thinking. Cultivating these skills and becoming adept at applying them is what we term *ethical competency*. The skills of ethical competency cannot be taught as a procedure, though it is possible that methods or conceptual devices can be utilized as aids in reasoning and decision-making. The skills of ethical competency are better thought of as skills that you would learn in a similar fashion to the way you learn to become proficient in an art.

Ethical competency is a creative skill set. This view has appeal when we think of the task of ethics as a practice of doing good. Through your ethical action, you create opportunities for the growth of your own integrity. You sow the possibility of growth for others around you and help to create a more positive social environment.

As a creative skill set, developing ethical skills is primarily a matter of practice. The best way to learn ethical skill is by doing. Aristotle noted that the practice of ethics is a practice of developing habits (Aristotle, 2002, pp. 21–23). This point is given a bit of style by Will Durant: "We are what we repeatedly do" (Durant, 1933, p. 87). The cultivation of habits is not a matter of mindless doing. We are, all of us, complex learners. We can draw from instruction from observation of these skills in others (role models). We can employ exercises to develop and test skills. We can consciously think about the art we practice (ethics) and the skills needed to practice it. As we identify these skills, we can think more about them, develop ideas about how to apply them, and think about cases and situations in which they apply. We can, in short, do some philosophical work with these skills. Think about what ethical competency is. Think about what it is like to be ethically competent. And do more than think about it. Wonder. Practice. Bring this to your life. The real philosophical work is in bringing these skills to your moral world.

THE SKILLS OF ETHICAL COMPETENCY

There are several skills that we can identify as part of ethical competency. These skills enable us to perform the various core tasks of moral agency. As an ethically competent person, you will be able to clarify moral issues, take on different perspectives, adjust your perspective as needed, gain a sense of direction in a difficult issue, and develop your sense of self and belonging in your social world. All of this will involve reasoning skills. Because you already encounter the world through your own moral reactions, your ethical reasoning will need to acknowledge and explore these reactions. You also have a set of moral beliefs that are informed by your culture, your upbringing, people around you, your personal experiences, as well as by your moral reactions. Your reasoning will need to account for, and explore, these also. Your reactions and beliefs are limited. Your reasoning will have to employ skills at fact gathering.

Your ethical competency takes place at an intersection of your reactions, background beliefs, and circumstances. You find yourself in a situation that requires your ethical attention and skill. A lot has met you there. Ethical competency means making use of the skills that will help you bring productive attention to this intersection.

Skills for ethical competency include skills in gathering facts, building perspective, and critical thinking. The skills you learn in performing an assessment will serve you in other areas of your life. They apply to your moral agency as well (Ferrell & Coyle, 2008). Don't rely on your initial assumptions. Carefully scrutinize the situation you face. Take note of the people who are involved. Identify the issue and the perspectives of the different people involved in this situation. If there is some charge of wrongdoing, determine exactly what the charge is and investigate to see if the available facts support this charge. Pay attention. Be as careful and as thorough as you can be in gathering facts.

Part of **gathering facts** is taking note of the perspectives of other people. You acknowledge what stances people take, what opinions they offer, and what solutions they propose. As you build perspective, you explore these viewpoints more carefully. Try to be open to the viewpoints of others. What reasons can they give for the view they take? Whether or not you initially agree with this viewpoint can you approach it with a charitable and open mind? Can you see a different viewpoint as a viable alternative?

A crucial part of **building perspective** is acknowledging that you come into this moral situation with a perspective of your own. Identify your own intuitive reaction to the situation. What are you feeling? What is your initial description of the event? You already know that this reaction of yours is a viable perspective—you have demonstrated its viability by possessing it yourself. Can you be open to the possibility that you can take a different viewpoint? Can you see the opportunity to change your mind if needed?

How do you know if you can change your mind? How do you know when you should change your mind? What makes a change of mind possible in the first place? This is where critical thinking comes in.

Gathering facts is a set of skills in ethical competency entailing the ability to objectively and thoroughly assess a moral situation.

Building perspective is a set of skills in ethical competency entailing the ability to consider different viewpoints with an open and charitable mind.

CRITICAL THINKING

The ideal critical thinker is habitually inquisitive, well-informed, trustful of reason, open-minded, flexible, fair-minded in evaluation, honest in facing personal biases, prudent in making judgments, willing to reconsider, clear about issues, orderly in complex matters, diligent in seeking relevant information, reasonable in the selection of criteria, focused in inquiry, and persistent in seeking results which are as precise as the subject and the circumstances of inquiry permit. Source: Facione (1990).

Ethical thinking is an application of critical thinking. In a health-care setting, *critical* has certain connotations that might be distracting when we wish to describe a kind of thinking as "critical." When we speak of critical care, for instance, we are talking about trauma or multisystem organ failure. The critical health state is a state of dependence. The patient is not stable, and the situation must be managed. In critical care, everything depends on swift and sure decision-making.

Critical thinking is important. It is not always life and death. *Critical*, in this usage, refers to the act of offering an evaluation and an analysis. Critical thinking is an examination, a critique.

The main work of critical thinking is the careful and rigorous sorting out of alternative perspectives. The aim of critical thinking is to undertake a deep examination of facts and interpretations and perspectives. The critical thinker is looking for insight into what is happening, what goals are worth pursuing, and for ways to pursue those goals (Chan, 2013; Dewey, 1998).

Fact gathering is essential to critical thinking. The analysis you undertake is best when you have reliable, accurate, and complete information. Think of what needs to happen in an assessment. You need to know what's going on. Opinions and reactions aren't going to be enough.

Critical thinking tests different options and interpretations. The facts need to be looked at from different angles. Finding the best goal means entertaining different ideas about what goals are worthwhile and what makes them worthwhile. Finding the best advice for the pursuit of goals means considering several options.

Consider the difference between critical thinking and *uncritical thinking*. Thinking that is uncritical will be quick to accept an idea without stopping for reflection. In the heart/hand/head model, the uncritical thinker will operate either on the basis of the heart's intuition or on the basis of the orders given to the hand alone. Uncritical thinking is easier inasmuch as it takes less time or because it readily conforms to prevailing views. It is easier, but it can be misinformed. Uncritical thinking closes the mind and prevents us from potentially finding better views, better ideas, and strategies to attain better outcomes (Dewey, 1998).

Critical thinking is a process of reasoned analysis aimed at arriving at a sound judgment. The critical thinker is challenged to seek out and take into account evidence, new information, and differing perspectives. The critical thinker takes all this information and makes evaluations by making careful inferences.

Critical thinking is reflective. The critical thinker acknowledges the appeal of heart and hand and takes them seriously. Thinking critically, you consider what you feel. You think about the orders that you have been given. You investigate, you ponder, you delve into these orders. Why do you feel this way? What other options are available? In what way do these orders make sense? What options do you have within the parameters of your orders?

Recognize what critical thinking does. It takes on perspectives and investigates them. It picks up arguments, ideas, and proposals and turns them over. It takes careful notice of ideas, becomes familiar with them, and appreciates them for what they are. It tests them to see if they hold up to scrutiny.

Imagine that you stop at a vendor's fruit stand. You want to buy one piece of fruit from a bin that holds dozens. You want something that fits your standards for ripeness, texture, and flavor. You can't actually taste each piece of fruit in the bin, but you don't have to just grab a piece at random. Pick one up and take note of how it looks, how it feels, and how it smells. Put that one down and pick up another one that looks to be a likely candidate for what you need. Repeat. This is a process of critical evaluation. Now, do this with ideas, arguments, and proposals.

Critical thinking works with options. It might be that critical thinking sorts through strategic options for practical action. It is always the case that critical thinking sorts through options for viewing and interpreting. Even if you have no choice about how to act, you have choices about how to view and understand the situation in which you act. You have choices about how to view yourself as a professional and as a moral agent.

There is a difference between critical thinking and problem solving. They are not opposed; critical thinking can often be of great use in problem solving. However, they are not identical. You can solve a problem, like a puzzle, without engaging critical thinking. Moreover, critical thinking does not promise that you will arrive at the right answer. The aim of critical thinking is to gain *insight*. The process of holding ideas in a new light, of gaining new perspectives aims at discovery. This discovery is not just a new vantage point, but a deeper and better way of seeing. Answers might come to you as you take this vantage point, but the vantage point itself has benefits.

Ethics, like critical thinking, is a *process*. Moral intuitions are states—conditions describing a momentary interaction between you and a given circumstance. Ethics is a process that utilizes some degree of careful deliberation in which you pursue this interaction in more depth. The goal is not just to have a reaction, but to determine how you should act, what you should value, what your role is, and who you ought to be.

ASSESSMENT/INTERVENTION/EVALUATION

Throughout human history, it has been persistently observed that many people would rather not put in the work involved in thinking critically. Even when you don't have a clear reaction to a moral challenge, you still might not want to invest the effort into a careful deliberation that will bring you to a decision about right and wrong. Often, we look for fast (and sloppy) ways to evade the demands of ethical inquiry—relying on authority, relying on tradition, relying on our intuitions and relying on our feelings.

However, think about it, these shortcuts to avoid thinking through a moral problem are entirely unacceptable elsewhere in your professional training. In a clinical setting, for instance, critical thinking is expected as part of doing your job and properly caring for your patients.

Nurses are trained to assess, do an intervention, and then evaluate. This same pattern applies to ethical inquiry as well. It's not really that hard. What makes ethical inquiry challenging is that you sometimes have to exert the effort to question and modulate your moral intuition. In addition, the circumstances in which you have to apply ethical inquiry can be challenging and ambiguous. You might not know what to do, but that's why you're assessing.

MORAL AGENCY

Ethics isn't just about feelings and beliefs. It's about participation. You are an active participant in the world. You belong to a world with other people with whom you interact in ways that can influence your sense of value. You face circumstances in this world that contribute to the conditions of your life. You recognize that you face choices regarding the way you interact with others and the way you address circumstances. What you do matters. The choices you make matter. The perspective you take matters. How you modulate your intuitions matters.

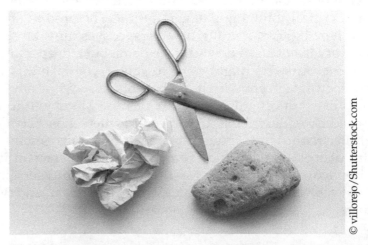

© villorejo/Shutterstock.com

Figure 2.1

Ethics is a way to look at value: specifically, the value that you bring—or fail to bring—to your social world through your actions. A moral agent is someone who has the potential to bring value through choices that the agent makes. This means you.

Ethics is social; there is always room to grow as an individual and with other people. Ethics is a process, not an achievement. Saying *I'm an ethical person, I don't need to study this or analyze it* is like saying *I've eaten already. I don't need to eat ever again.*

A **moral agent**—like you—possesses the capacity to identify circumstances in which there is something at stake morally. A moral agent also recognizes that there is something significant at stake in making choices about how to act. The choices you make and the way you act matters. Through your actions, you can cause harm, avoid harm, or alleviate harm. You can foster or share joy. There is value at stake in what you do. Hence, the moral agent acknowledges responsibility for choices made and for actions that are intended to follow those choices.

Free will coincides with moral expectations. We recognize that ethics places some restrictions on what we freely choose to do. We also recognize that part of free will is the free choice to restrain and guide your own actions according to moral value.

Humility is an important component of moral agency. As a critical thinker, it is helpful to have the humility to realize that you don't have all the answers right in front of you. You have work to do in order to sort out possible options. You need the humility to realize that your intuitions might not be your best guide, and that other people might have a perspective that is worth your time. Humility expands the freedom of your will by opening space for wonder and new ideas.

Your humility will also be useful as you identify the difference between what you can do and what you can't do. You are able to exercise your agency in order to have an impact on the world. Yet you know that you cannot take authority over everything that happens. Other people are moral agents, too. We are all subject to circumstances beyond our control. As a moral agent, you face some limits in the influence you can have. It is also possible to surrender authority that you could legitimately exercise. Moral agents don't make choices or accept responsibility everywhere that they could. Sometimes, the will is only constrained by lack of use.

We can say of a moral agent that some behaviors or experiences will be *agential* or *nonagential*. A moral agent who embraces agency—that is, accepts that a choice must be made and that there is some responsibility for making this choice—is acting agentially. All other behaviors or experiences will be nonagential. This includes failing to recognize that a choice can be made or that there is responsibility for this choice. Recognizing that there is a choice, but not making it is also nonagential.

You act agentially when you realize that you face a choice that will have impact. Think of those moments when you recognized that something of moral worth depended on your choice and that you should

Moral agent is a person who can make a decision to act in one's social world and who recognizes some responsibility to make those choices in a way that can be recognized as "right".

Humility as a moral quality, humility is the recognition that your moral value is not greater than anyone else's and that your moral beliefs might not contain all the answers.

make this choice with ethical skill. At that moment, you saw that your choice mattered. You were agential in that moment.

FOR WHOM DO I MAKE A DIFFERENCE?

Take a moment to answer the question that titles this section. For whom do you make a difference? Who do you have obligations toward?

What questions do you want answered before you can answer this question? How does your answer change depending on whether you are talking about your professional life or your personal life? What about making a difference for complete strangers that you never expect to see again? Once more, does it matter if we are talking about professional interaction or an encounter with a stranger on the street?

The point is that your participation matters for many people and in different ways. Let's consider three main arenas in which you can make a difference.

CATEGORIES

Think about the difference you can make as an upstanding member of your profession, as an employee, or as a proud graduate of your academic program. You can make a difference for humanity in general. You can, in other words, make a difference for people gathered together according to some (more or less) abstract categorization.

We can speak of duties to humanity. (Indeed, we will in the next chapter.) Such duties are based on abstract notions of human nature, personhood, respect, and rights. Though we are all unique individually, we speak of humanity as sharing elements in common.

The abstract nature of the categories we draw matches the ephemeral way in which we might be said to make a difference. What does it mean, after all, to make a difference for humanity as a whole?

GROUPS

The categories we draw are abstractions. On a practical level, we gather into social groupings—families, networks of friends, co-workers, and so on. We find here that we can make a difference for a specific group. The members of this group are bound together in some practical way. Actions that benefit the members of this group benefit the group as a whole in some way.

Because of the nature of the group, you might be able to benefit someone without directly interacting with a specific person. You can have an impact on people by helping to shape procedures that others will follow, by mentoring someone whose actions will improve because of your instruction. You might be in position to see your impact on the group even though some members of the group might not know of the difference you made on their behalf.

RELATIONAL

On a personal perspective, there are people for whom you can directly make a difference. Family members and friends all connect with you in intimate, personal ways. You also connect interpersonally with coworkers, professors, students. Sometimes strangers can connect with you as you offer a helping hand or engage in conversation on a bus. Your work with patients will be here.

Thinking of categories and groups, it is possible to act in such a way that your ethical competency is not fully noticed even though it may have considerable impact. In a relational arena, your ethical competency is noticed. The way you interact with people on an individual basis is noticeable to that person. You are right there, sharing the same space.

EXERCISE

Think about how these arenas apply to your professional work. In what way will your profession bring you into direct contact with another person? In what ways will you have impact on groups or entire categories?

WHY BE ETHICAL? ETHICAL COMPETENCY AND THE ART OF BEING HUMAN

Many philosophers argue that practice in ethics enhances your humanity. They argue that ethical competency contributes in several ways to living a better life. The good life. A life of significance.

Exercising your moral skills can mean making choices that involve sacrifice of your own pleasure or well-being. Sometimes the exercise of moral skills is hard. What you realize is the right choice isn't always the easy choice or the one that will give you pleasure. However, knowing that you've made the right choice or that you've brought about some good for someone else might give you some sort of satisfaction. This satisfaction is described by philosopher Immanuel Kant as a way of being worthy of happiness.

Ethical competency may be essential to living up to the expectations of your social and professional roles. This social and professional competency can bring personal rewards as well as harmony in your encounters with others at work and in your society. Your commitment to ethics can help you be more effective in your profession. These skills can help you to see your circumstances with greater clarity and to develop an improved sense of priority. You are in better position to bring about better outcomes.

Acting with ethical competency can bring personal and social benefits. The listening and caring skills that position you to act with kindness and fairness toward others can have the effect of encouraging others to act with kindness and fairness toward you. We call this **reciprocity**. This isn't necessarily a promise that the good you do for others will be returned to you in equal measure, but we do see a tendency in people to think more favorably of those they regard as exhibiting prosocial behaviors.

Reciprocity is a mutual exchange of like for like. It can be thought of as a matter of merit in which good is rewarded with good and bad is punished with bad. Or, it can describe an interpersonal connection in which a caring gesture by one person toward another helps both people mutually.

Many philosophers argue that ethical competency is an essential component of happiness. Distinct from pleasure, happiness as an ethical matter is seen as a long-term condition. The happy person has reached a state of self-assurance. The happy person is in a continual state of self-improvement—not perfected but striving to become better. That sense of striving itself brings freshness, a novelty, to one's sense of self. Moral skills can moderate excesses of emotion and ego-driven impulses. Morality makes your life a little less about you. Paradoxically, this works out better for you as you are better able to enjoy enriched and healthy relationships.

It won't be the case that the exercise of your moral skills will encourage absolutely everyone to act morally toward you. For instance, your moral behavior might be taken by others as a sign of weakness. In another paradox, moral skill can also provide the capacity to endure hardship and see a way to respond appropriately to unfairness and injustice without giving away your sense of self.

There is satisfaction that comes from knowing that your actions have moral worth. The foregoing survey comes back to a fundamental concern for harm. Why be ethical? It helps you to avoid doing harm and, when it can't be entirely avoided, to bring about the best outcomes possible in the midst of it.

FROM SIMPLICITY TO COMPLEXITY

Normative ethics is that branch of philosophical ethics that examines questions about how one ought to act and who one ought to be.

In Chapter 1, you were introduced to the difference between your moral feelings and ethical assessment. Ethical assessment can be related to a clinical model of inquiry in which we follow the stages assessment/intervention/evaluation. We develop this connection further here. The task ahead of us in this chapter is to explore what is involved in the process of ethical assessment and evaluation. In the next chapter, we will explore ethical inquiry as it can be informed by **normative ethical** theory. Theory can be used to attain a plan for an intervention when your involved in a situation that requires a moral decision.

Recall also the attention in Chapter 1 to harm as a guiding idea in health-care ethics. The process of ethical thinking can be viewed as way to assess situations in which moral harm is at stake. This assessment arrives at an intervention—a course of action that seems best suited to bringing about benefit while avoiding undue harm. As the intervention is taken, ethical thinking continues to monitor the situation to determine if the intervention actually works as hoped and to see if better options become apparent.

It's one thing to talk about making ethical decisions. It's quite another to examine how it's done. We've already established that critical thinking is part of the process of thinking ethically. But, here again, advocating critical thinking isn't the same as explaining how it's done. Are you sighing? It's understandable.

Let's start with a nod to what we all have experienced: Moral situations are challenging. There is no set way to defeat ethical conundrums by finding a magic key that unlocks its mysteries. Then again, ethics really isn't that hard most of the time. Most of the time, you act properly with full confidence that you know what to do. Such is your confidence that you probably aren't even recognizing the ethical implications of the situation you face or the action you choose in that situation. You meet a patient for the first time; you don't intend to cause any harm. Good for you; that's the ethical choice! You follow the protocol for hand washing before you touch a patient. Maybe you recognize the importance of this safety protocol, but did you think about the ethical implications of the protocol? As you prepare an injection to administer to a patient, you listen and respond as the patient chatters nervously. How do you view your act? Do you think about the ethics involved in listening to this patient? If we're honest, we'll all probably recognize that most of the time, we pay little attention to ethics. We're busy, after all. We tend to treat morality as something we only need to worry about under certain circumstances. Often, this view seems to be right.

For the most part, our moral feelings really are effective guides to action. It seems to be our tendency to avoid causing harm. We also show a tendency to identify the intentional causation of harm as a problem to be addressed and corrected.

In 2015, Niels Högel, a nurse in Germany, was sentenced on two counts each of murder and attempted murder. Working in critical care units, Högel would inject drugs into a patient in order to initiate cardiac arrest. Högel claimed that he wanted to see if he could resuscitate the patient. Very often, he couldn't. In 2017, it was announced that further investigations turned up evidence that Högel had murdered at least 100 people.

There is no question that Högel's deeds were reprehensible. Ethically, these actions cannot be defended. There is a clear intent to needlessly cause harm. Högel placed vulnerable patients on a trajectory toward death that they otherwise would not have followed at that time. Worse, Högel was a professional charged with the care of these patients.

First, do no harm. Högel violated that adage to a monstrous degree.

EXERCISE

Was Högel monstrous? How would you describe what makes actions monstrous in terms of ethics? Can we arrive at a simple answer? What does your attempt at an answer say about your expectations regarding our natural capacity to be good people?

FOUR VITAL INTENTIONS

We're back to the root of health-care ethics—the avoidance of harm. We've seen that, strictly speaking, avoiding harm doesn't fully cover all of our moral concerns. This would hold the bar for ethical behavior too low. Consider the opposite of Högel's case—a nurse in a critical care unit who does not inject medications into a patient for the purpose of initiating cardiac arrest. Can you imagine this? Of course you can. This happens every day, in every critical care unit, everywhere. Most of the time, you act properly. It is part of your normal conduct that you avoid causing harm. While it is good of you to avoid causing needless harm as you go through your day, this is such a basic expectation that it will not single you out as being particularly worthy of praise. *Do no harm* is really a starting point. Ethically, we might want more. As living beings, we all have the capacity to grow. Harm obstructs growth, and the avoidance of harm can allow the conditions for growth to be utilized. But we also need some attention to establishing the conditions for growth. As social beings, we need the assistance of others in relationship with us to aid in establishing conditions for growth. Sometimes we need more from others than to refrain from harming us. On many occasions and in many ways, we need people to be willing to show up for us.

> *First, do no harm.*
> *Be willing.*

Understand that these adages are little more than catchphrases. The sum of ethics cannot be found just by repeating these. However, in these, we find a first look at the core of what we want from ethics. Putting these adages together allows us to affirm four vital intentions:

1. *Where there is suffering, do not add harm. (Do no harm, version 1)*
2. *Where there is suffering, do what you can to alleviate it.*
3. *Where there is no suffering, do not add harm. (Do no harm, version 2)*
4. *Where there is no suffering, maintain and nurture what is good.*

We see something close to these intentions in the preamble of the Code of Ethics published by the International Council of Nurses: "Nurses have four fundamental responsibilities: to promote health, to prevent illness, to restore health and to alleviate suffering" (ICN, 2012). The responsibility to alleviate suffering clearly aligns with the second of the vital intentions: "Where there is suffering, do what you can to alleviate it". It would seem that this intention is also reflected in the responsibility to restore health. Counseling people about hygiene, immunizations, nutrition, exercise, and lifestyle choices are ways to promote health. These efforts cultivate good where there may be no suffering. Measures that fit within a culture of safety—such as hand-washing, taking measures to prevent falls, checking for allergies—are efforts to prevent illness and injury. These are ways to actively seek to avoid adding harm that does not presently exist. These measures are undertaken in a clinical environment that is populated by people who are already suffering under other conditions. Therefore, the responsibility to prevent illness describes both versions of *do no harm*.

FOUR VITAL INTENTIONS	
Where there is suffering, do not add harm. *Prevent illness and injury*	Where there is no suffering, do not add harm. *Prevent illness and injury*
Where there is suffering, do what you can to alleviate it. *Alleviate suffering and restore health*	Where there is no suffering, maintain and nurture what is good. *Promote health*

Figure 2.2 Four Intentions Table

These intentions quickly present possible complications and conflicts. Causing harm is bad, but what if some harm needs to be caused in order to address the source of someone's suffering? For instance, an incision causes pain, but this is deemed acceptable when a surgical procedure is the best course of action to address certain conditions. Asking one person to donate a kidney to another poses the risk of creating harm where there was none in order to address the suffering for another. While our moral feelings are often effective behavioral guides, the possibility of complicated scenarios may be the source of confusion among our intentions. Ethics becomes complicated. It is tempting to suggest that it is when we reach complications in which our moral feelings are ill-equipped to guide us intuitively that *ethics* properly emerges. At the least, it is in these situations in which we are confused, lost, frustrated, or distressed that ethical assessment is especially necessary.

LEVELS OF ETHICAL ASSESSMENT

There is another source of complication to our ethical thinking. This complication is inherent within our capacity for ethical thinking itself. Look again at the four vital intentions. Do not create harm where none exists. This is a nice sentiment, and rather clear. But how are we to respect this? Do we avoid causing needless harm by establishing laws to prohibit such acts, or write policies and procedures in order to steer people away from acts of harm? Should we carefully identify possible harms we might cause and then plan our actions so that we can avoid them? Is it good to get to know people such that we can tell how they are vulnerable and act toward them with a sensibility to avoid exploiting those vulnerabilities?

The answer to all those questions is potentially *Yes*. These questions are not inherently at odds. Depending on circumstances, it may be possible to address each one of them and arrive at a coherent view of how we should act. In such a case, it might even be that one way of addressing the question will be so compelling as to make the other questions rather irrelevant in comparison. Moreover, we might find that the answer we derive from asking one question is not entirely consistent with the answers derived from other questions. Still, all of these are legitimate and useful ways of ethically inquiring into how we should act.

These questions correspond to three main levels of ethical assessment. The first way of questioning aligns with an *administrative* level of assessment in which we seek principles, policies, and laws that offer standards that all should respect. The second way of questioning aligns with a *strategic* level of assessment in which we seek a practical solution for a specific moral situation. Here, we examine possible courses of action in search of the one that holds the promise of bringing about the best outcomes. The third way of questioning aligns with an *interpersonal* level of assessment in which one is present with someone of moral value whose suffering, or potential suffering, commands one's attention.

The next step is to take a closer look at each level on an individual basis. The next chapter will account for some of the practical ways in which you already engage each level of thinking. To deepen your examination, and to help provide a means to further clarify moral issues, each level of ethical assessment will be explored from a theoretical angle. All of this will be brought together in Chapter 3 as an Ethical Assessment Model.

EXERCISE

As you approach this book and your study of ethics, be open to the process of developing ethical skills. You already have these. This book is intended to offer practice, information, ideas, and, above all, perspective. Critical thinking is not the whole of ethics, but it is essential to the process. It is a necessary skill.

Critical thinking isn't problem solving. The exercises and case studies in this book are not set up to challenge you to find the right answers. For some exercises and case studies, there might be answers that are clearly right. For all of them, the benefit is in the critical exploration and in the opportunity to work with ideas. Open yourself to the exploration. Engage everything here as an exercise in thought and wonder. We are talking about important topics—the welfare of your patients, your professional career, and your integrity. The insight you gain—from this book and everywhere you turn your critical attention—will serve you well in your moral world.

REFERENCES

Aristotle. (2002). *Nicomachean ethics.* (J. Sachs, Trans.) Newbury, MA: Focus Pub./R. Pullins.

ASCT. (2006). *Guidelines for the ethical practice of cytotechnology.* American Society for Cytotechnology. Retrieved from http://www.asct.com/docs/Guidelines_for_the_Ethical_Practice_of_Cytotechnology_approved.pdf

Chan, Z. C. Y. (2013). A systematic review of critical thinking in nursing education. *Nurse Education Today* 33(3): 236–240.

Dewey, J. (1998). *How we think: A restatement of the relation of reflective thinking to the educative process.* Chicago, IL: Henry Regnery Company.

Durant, W. (1933). *The story of philosophy.* Garden City, NY: Garden City Publishing Co., Inc.

Facione, P. A. (1990). Consensus statement regarding critical thinking and the ideal critical thinker. In *Critical thinking: A statement of expert consensus for purposes of educational assessment and instruction: Executive Summary: The Delphi report.* Millbrae, CA: The California Academic Press.

Ferrell, B. R., & Coyle, N. (2008). *The nature of suffering and the goals of nursing.* New York: Oxford University Press.

ICN. (2012). *The ICN code of ethics for nurses.* Geneva, Switzerland: International Council of Nurses. Retrieved from http://www.icn.ch/images/stories/documents/about/icncode_english.pdf

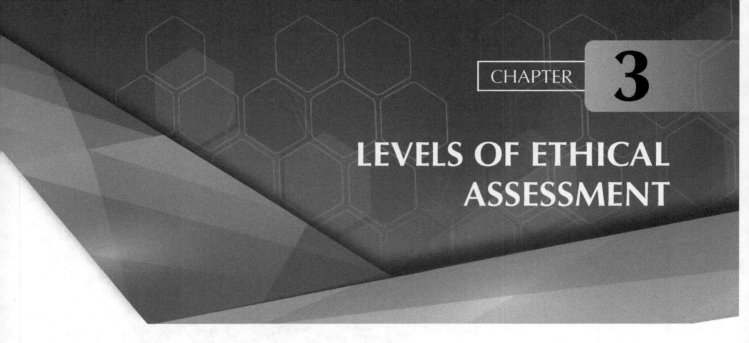

CHAPTER 3

LEVELS OF ETHICAL ASSESSMENT

OBJECTIVES

After completing this chapter, you will be able to . . .

1. Describe the three levels of ethical assessment: administrative, strategic, and interpersonal.

2. Understand the relevance of policy and regulation in administrative-level thinking.

3. Understand and utilize the principle of biomedical ethics and the categorical imperative in administrative-level ethical assessment.

4. Understand the relevance of procedure and protocol in strategic-level thinking.

5. Understand and utilize utilitarianism in strategic-level ethical assessment.

6. Identify the difference between empathy and compassion as guides to ethical action.

7. Understand the relevance of narrative in interpersonal-level thinking.

8. Understand and utilize compassion in interpersonal-level ethical assessment.

9. Apply the Ethical Assessment Model as a means to explore a moral issue.

KEY TERMS

- Administrative-level ethical assessment
- Authentic presence
- Categorical imperative
- Compassion
- Consequentialism
- Deontology
- Humanity formulation of the categorical imperative

- Interpersonal-level ethical assessment
- Maxim
- Narrative
- Negative rights
- Positive rights

- Principles
- Rights
- Strategic-level ethical assessment
- Utilitarianism
- Willingness

Principle 1

....

The Nuclear Medicine Technologist will provide services with compassion and respect for the dignity of the individual and with the intent to provide the highest quality of patient care (NMTCB, 2012).

THE LEVELS OF ETHICAL ASSESSMENT

Administrative-level ethical assessment focuses on rights and principles that apply to all members of broad category (such as humanity). This level aligns with deontological ethical theories.

The three levels of assessment are key to engaging in a full ethical assessment. The presentation of these levels is intended to draw attention to the wide reach and scope of ethics. This chapter will lead to a model for assessment that utilizes these three levels. The model is not intended to make ethics easy or simple. It is intended to serve as a guide and as a reminder. Ethical analysis involves challenges. You'll need to identify your own moral reactions and critically analyze them. You'll need to acknowledge that other people have moral reactions of their own. As you build perspective using the three levels of assessment, you'll find new ways to challenge and explore these reactions. In the process, insight can develop and ideas for effective and compassionate action can emerge.

THREE LEVELS OF ETHICAL ASSESSMENT		
Administrative	**Strategic**	**Interpersonal**
Standards for everyone to follow; determination of groups with special concerns	Assess possible outcomes for desirability and cost	Therapeutic compassion and authentic presence
Appropriate action is consistent with principles and policies	Appropriate action is the most promising route to the best possible outcome	Appropriate action is a combination of authentic presence and actions responsive to the needs of the person

Figure 3.1 Three Levels of Ethical Assessment

Consider a hospital. Policies and procedures are established at an **administrative level** in order to ensure compliance with established legal, professional, and financial standards. Administration is at some distance from actual patient care and only impacts that care by establishing proscriptive and prescriptive boundaries that guide the actions and decisions of those who deliver care. Policies are general, applying across the board to all people who enter the hospital or to people who are broadly categorized into a group (e.g., patients, visitors, employees).

Decisions about patient care are made on a strategic level. Treatment decisions are made on the basis of careful attention to the patient's major complaint, medical history, physical workup, and evidence from diagnostic tests. The differential diagnosis is a systematic process to identify the problem. This process may involve several people including the physician, the patient, radiologists and other members of the medical team, and members of the patient's family. Once a diagnosis is made, options for treatment are considered and evaluated. Treatment follows according to the assessment/intervention/evaluation model. This strategic level is aimed at promoting the best possible health outcome for the patient.

At the **strategic level**, decisions are made about what interventions will be offered to a patient. In other words, the strategic level determines what care is offered. A nurse might have orders to administer a certain medication. A radiology tech might have orders to perform a specific scan. Such orders determine actions that are to be performed in pursuit of desired outcomes for the patient. How those actions are performed; what sort of interaction occurs between the medical professional and the patient also have importance. How that care is given falls under the interpersonal level. This level is immediate and intimate. It is an opportunity to affirm that worth of the person you encounter—be it a patient or a coworker.

The **interpersonal level** is the place of encounter. Space is shared with someone else: perhaps a patient under your care, a family member who is in the room, or a coworker. What happens in this interaction? What occurs in this space? These interactions can be constrained by demands on your time or the attention demanded by the task you have to perform. Still, there is the question of how this interaction goes. Do you have the willingness to affirm the person with whom you interact? Can you be present? Can you listen? Can this interaction be an occasion for compassion?

The image of the hospital just given has taken three different perspectives. The administrative level is the furthest removed from patient care, yet its purview has the broadest reach over all of the hospital's stakeholders. The strategic level occurs at the level of diagnosis and treatment plan. The work of health care happens here. The interpersonal level zooms in on this work, focusing on specific interactions and specific moments. All of these are important and of interest to us ethically. All of them potentially bear on the moral situations that we face and must make decisions about. As we can understand that a hospital needs all three of these levels for the effective delivery of health care, so we will pursue a multileveled approach to effective ethical assessment.

Strategic-level ethical assessment focuses on bringing about the best outcomes. This level aligns with consequentialist ethical theories, such as utilitarianism.

Interpersonal-level ethical assessment focuses on establishing strong and healthful relationships among persons. This level aligns with ethics of care and ethics of compassion.

We have the vital intentions to do no harm, to take care not to add needlessly to already existing suffering, to alleviate suffering where we can, and to go further to nurture conditions for good. Consider the subtle shadings in how we see these intentions from these different levels. At the administrative level, we are looking to set general rules to guide people away from harmful behaviors. At the strategic level, we are analyzing plans of action according to the likelihood that they will yield harm or benefit. Relationships are manifest at the interpersonal level. In this contact, there is witness to suffering and personal opportunity to alleviate suffering and to nurture conditions for good.

These levels of assessment are not mutually exclusive. They can be used in concert to develop needed perspective as you face a moral issue. We can, for instance, find that the principles we explain have an eye toward bringing about good outcomes. We can also find that fostering interpersonal connection is an important way of treating people with dignity and respect. At the same time, these different levels of assessment are not always going to speak as one. Depending on circumstances, they can sometimes be at tension with each other. Respecting someone's autonomy might mean supporting a patient's right to make a decision that is not conducive to the best outcomes for that patient.

These different levels of assessment are vantage points. Use them to enhance your view of a situation and your options. Bear in mind that you are a moral agent. Your participation in this world—and in your role as a health-care professional—matters. The levels of ethical assessment provide viewpoints from which to enhance your understanding of what you can do to address the problem of suffering.

Recall from Chapter 1 the passage from Śāntideva's *The Way of the Boddhisatva*:

> *For all those ailing in the world,*
> *Until their every sickness has been healed,*
> *May I myself become for them*
> *The doctor, nurse, the medicine itself. Source:* Śāntideva (2008, p. 48).

The three levels of ethical assessment are illustrated in this passage's appeal to the healing power of doctor, nurse, and medicine. The medicine has been developed without regard for a specific patient. Rather, it has been developed according to known properties of illness types, biochemical principles, and clinical trials on categories of test subjects. The doctor is the one who diagnoses, prescribes and treats, all in an effort to identify the suffering of a patient in order to bring about a better health outcome. The nurse is at the bedside providing care. This is the interpersonal level.

As we further explore each level of assessment, pay attention to how you already make use of it and how you can engage it with more depth. Keep in mind as well that each level is offered here as part of a larger process. Working in one level in your ethical assessment can help you as you work in the other levels.

The art of ethical competency involves developing skill at each of these levels. Developing this skill enables you to approach a given moral issue with perspective. You will be able to better grasp the positions taken by others and to draw from their insights. You will enhance and expand your vision. With humility, you will be able to offer your own moral agency with the informed intentions to do no harm and to show up.

ADMINISTRATIVE LEVEL

The concern at the administrative level is to set standards for behavior. We are looking to set general rules to guide people away from harmful behaviors and toward behaviors that promote human rights and dignity. The aim is to establish boundaries. Lines are drawn, delineating acceptable behavior from prohibited behavior. The standards set in this effort tend to be general and abstract. These standards are targeted, not to particular individuals in specific circumstances, but to categories of people. As they apply to categories of people, these standards are not specific guidelines of conduct, but broader in scope.

ALREADY IN PRACTICE

Policies, regulations, and laws establish general standards for behavior. While these are not necessarily the same as ethical standards, we will see that there can be an overlap between these standards and ethics. There can be an ethical element to observing policy and regulation.

In a way, some ethical decisions are already made for us at the administrative level. Many policies and regulations are intended to forestall harmful acts. While these policies and regulations might not always be legislated primarily for ethical reasons—providing protection against legal liability can be a powerful motivator—they nonetheless serve a role in guiding action for those subject to the policies.

There is a certain efficiency to this moral guidance provided by administrative policies. Moreover, indeed, administrative level of ethical assessment also promises efficiency. Once you have determined what your duties are, they establish a dependable presence. You know your duty. You might have to think about how a duty applies given the situation you face, and you might have to find the will to follow your duty, but the question of what your moral obligation is has been taken care of. Knowing your duty spares some time that would otherwise be spent looking for some kind of moral ground underneath your feet.

Time and effort are legitimate concerns for decision-making. Many of us feel too pressed for time to make thoughtful decisions. At least, that is a common complaint. In health-care, demands on time can, indeed, be severe. Efficiency in decision-making, therefore, is legitimately desirable. This is a prime reason for administrative level policies.

Policies are everywhere. Every place of employment has policies. A policy consists of a set of principles that guides decision-making. In addition to this set of guiding principles, a written policy may have a statement that defines the purpose for having the policy and objectives that are its goals. There may also be accounts of strategies to implement the policy and to measure its effectiveness and provisions that assign responsibilities to certain parties for carrying out and overseeing the policy. In addition, policies will often describe procedures that standardize actions to be taken in carrying out its core principles.

There is a distinction between policy and procedure. A policy is held over time to address a perceived need. Procedures are a detailed series of actions to be taken in order to serve the policy's purpose. A policy is effective over an extended period of time even though procedures mandated by those policies will only be used when warranted. Consider the insurance policy for a car. The policy states what kind of coverage you have on your car, including how much might be paid to the owner in the event of certain types of damage. If a claim has to be made, the policy dictates the procedure.

Policies and procedures may vary between organizations, but they are a valuable resource to ensure that regulations are followed. In health-care, policies and procedures are essential for standardizing practices that are in the spirit of avoiding harm. Health-care often has extensive policies covering issues from ethical practices, to occupational safety guidelines, to confidentiality—all within the duty to care.

Many regulatory agencies establish policies to set guidelines for behavior. In many cases, the prevention of harm is central to the purpose and operation of regulatory agencies. The policies they set, therefore, will seek to place boundaries around activities that involve a heightened risk for harm.

As an example, consider a policy that involves cleaning blood from a surface. The Occupational Safety and Health Administration under the United States Department of Labor (OSHA) offers guidelines and clean-up standards to protect workers (OSHA, n.d.). The Centers for Disease Control and Prevention (CDC) has an interest in preventing the transmission of blood-borne pathogens and provides management and treatment guidelines (NIOSH, 2018). OSHA regulations also require the United States Environmental Protection Agency (EPA) to develop an Exposure Control Plan to minimize the risk of occupational and environmental exposure of pathogens when spills are cleaned and cleaning materials are disposed (EPA, n.d.). The facility where the blood is cleaned will have a policy specific to their disposal process. Then, that disposed material needs to be transported to a disposal site and State departments of transportation will have regulations concerning this transference. Therefore, one policy involving clean-up of a blood spill will have to incorporate federal and state regulations, laws, and guidelines.

Policies can be set by government statue, by government agency, by a third-party industry regulatory agency, by a professional organization, and by a company or corporate entity. These policies can overlap and reinforce each other—as seen with the multiple regulations concerning blood-borne pathogens. Overlapping policies can also differ in specific ways, making attention to detail a challenge and, sometimes, a hassle.

While policies consist of principles, it is not the case that every policy consists of ethical principles. (We will explore the nature of ethical principles below.) The inspiration for a policy might not be a moral incentive to do good or avoid harm. Policies can be put in place as cost-saving measures, as protections against litigation, or in compliance with government regulations. Even so, many policies, regardless of the motivation behind them, do have ethical significance.

EXERCISE

Even if a policy is not motivated by a moral incentive, is there some ethical worth in following a policy? Find a policy at your job or at your school (anywhere, really—just find one) that does not appear on the surface to be oriented to the prevention of harm or the establishment of good. Is it the case that this policy has no bearing on ethics, or is there some ethical reason to follow this policy anyway? Use Figure 3.1 to help examine the policy.

REGULATION

We will tend to focus on policies as they are encountered in one's occupation. Hence, our attention to policies will generally be restricted to those encountered when working in health-care. Because there is some use in understanding why an organization has the policies they do, we need to note a few other sources of administrative-level rules. Regulations, laws, ordinances, and statutes are similar to policies in that they establish rules that impose boundaries or guidelines. We particularly encounter these as they are created by federal, state, and local governments or by government agencies. Many policies are made in compliance with regulations, laws, ordinances, and statutes.

Typically, these legal guidelines and boundaries are enforceable. Breaking the law or violating a regulation can be punished with fines, loss of licensure, or imprisonment. Through law, government can compel people to adjust their behaviors. For that matter, companies can use policies to compel employees to adjust their behavior. Policies can specify risks of job loss, docked pay, or notes in personnel files for noncompliance. There exist strong incentives to regard laws, policies, and duties that must be followed.

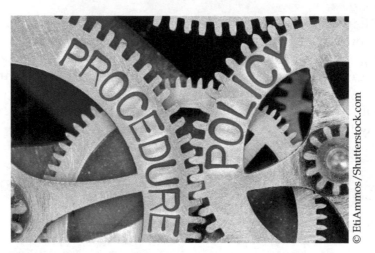

Figure 3.2

And so, we come to the difference between law (and regulations and statutes and such) and ethics. The interest in preventing undue harm is common to ethics and to law. Law functions by establishing guidelines.

Law is not intended to influence beliefs. Law only constrains or compels actions; it does not require that those who follow the law have any particular beliefs. You may, for instance, obey laws about paying your taxes whether or not you believe that the laws are just. In the same way, a policy at work doesn't require you to believe that the policy is a great idea. You are only required to believe that it is worthwhile to adhere to the policy. To act as a moral agent, however, assumes that you believe that the action you choose to perform is ethically justified. Put another way: The policies and regulations that are set for you by your employer and by government are established with the expectation that you will follow the rules. Ethics, on the other hand, is an activity in which you are your own legislator. That is, ethical competency means treating your moral agency as one who goes through a deliberate process of establishing the ethical rules by which you will live. It is this process of establishing such rules that is the administrative level of ethical assessment.

NORMATIVE THEORY

In the administrative level, ethical standards are often expressed as duties. Normative theories that focus on the ethical standards we draw at this level are often labeled *deontological*. From Greek roots, the term means *a study of duty*. Such an orientation means that deontology can have appeal as a very duty- or rule-based approach. It also means that deontology will tend to be very abstract as it recommends actions.

Deontology emphasizes rules and intentions. Imagine yourself in a moral situation. In deontology, you act rightly when you have your mind on two self-reflective questions: *What rules apply in this situation? What are my intentions?* Immediately, you'll see a curious thing: Your decision about how to act is not driven by questions that focus on this specific action. The choice of action should flow from deliberation over rules and duties. Ultimately, the concern is to focus on your mindset and outlook.

Rules are an administrative-level device for identifying and setting boundaries. They are rather like traffic signals that tell you where you may, and may not, go. Traffic signals help to standardize the movement of traffic, helping to foster an overall flow. This flow establishes some expectations for safety and relatively equitable level of convenience of travel for everyone.

Part of drawing boundaries involves placing people into categories. If this sounds overly bureaucratic, think of all the categories we commonly consider: Human, Citizen, Patients, Employees, and so on. Membership in these abstract categories often comes down to a small set of criteria, making membership determinations fairly straightforward: One is either a member of such-and-such a category or one is not. This makes it possible to lean on the concept of *equality* in the administrative level: All citizens are equal before the law. All patients deserve our best care. All humans are equal in their moral worth. This last example sits at the heart of standards in the administrative level. Equality of moral worth corresponds to notions of respect for all humanity and for the idea that we can look for moral duties that universally bind all human beings.

Seeing all humans as having equal moral value provides the grounds for practical use of the administrative level of ethical assessment. Think of this in terms of principles and rights. If all humans have equal moral value, then any moral principle that you want to hold as a good one to follow should be a good one for all humans to follow. If one human is entitled to a certain right, then it must be said that all humans are entitled to this same right, since all humans are all equal in worth.

The deontologist offers a perspective in which right action is not to be determined from outcomes that you anticipate or hope to see. Instead, right action is determined by your own commitment to rules that bring you to focus either on the rightness or wrongness of your own act or on your act as it rightly or wrongly impacts the moral value of another person. In the first, we are looking toward principles. In the second, we are looking toward rights.

Principles are fundamental guidelines to be used as a reference for determining courses of action. In Chapter 1, we explored the standards set by four principles: autonomy, nonmaleficence, beneficence, and

Deontology is a normative ethical theory that explores moral duty, typically in the form of principles, rights, and obligations.

A **principle** is a fundamental proposition that guides action.

A **right** is a moral entitlement.

Negative rights pertain to an entitlement that persons have not to be treated in certain ways.

Positive rights pertain to entitlements that persons have to make certain claims.

justice. In this chapter, we'll examine the use of these in making an ethical assessment.

We think of **rights** as a natural or acquired part of being a person with moral value. Having rights means that other people have duties toward you. Again, rights draw lines; these lines mark out what must not be done to you or what must be allowed for you. Some rights—those that mark what must not be done to you—are **negative rights**. These are strong proscriptions against actions in which other people would interfere with you. The right to autonomy is a negative right declaring that other people should not obstruct your capacity to choose. **Positive rights** mark goods or services that must be provided for you if you are to enjoy the dignity of personhood. In Chapter 10, we will explore the possibility of health-care as a positive right.

In deontology, avoiding unnecessary harm is recognized as a fundamental duty. Many of our ideas about rights stem from an observation about types of harm that should not be caused. Consider some of what we regard as negative rights—the right to life, right to free speech, and right to liberty. Notice what these rights claim: Innocent people are harmed if they are killed, so we should not violate their right to live. People are harmed if they are not allowed the opportunity to express their ideas. People are harmed if their capacity to live their lives as they choose is obstructed. This right to liberty has an obvious limitation: Your right to live as you choose ends at that point at which you would interfere with someone else's right to liberty. Which is to say that your right to liberty stops where you begin to cause harm to someone else.

If you don't see much difference between rights and principles, you needn't worry. The two tend to overlap. Indeed, the principle of autonomy is often expressed as a principle of *respect for autonomy,* implying a duty to respect someone's right to self-determination. If you have a right to determine the course of your own life, then others have an obligation to respect your autonomy. If others follow the principle of autonomy, then they are also respecting your right—and responsibility—to determine the course of your own life.

Immanuel Kant (1724–1804) is the philosopher best associated with deontological ethics. Kant sought to understand the rational basis of moral value, and he found it in autonomy. As noted in Chapter 1, autonomy literally means "self-rule." Self-rule describes individuals who legislate for themselves. Kant was not saying that ethics means making up your own moral rules or relying on your own opinions. The legislation he had in mind was the act

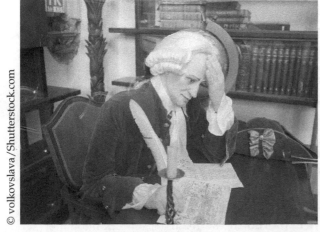

Figure 3.3 Immanuel Kant

of determining what the law *ought to be*; the act of thinking, reflecting, and discovering for yourself the moral law that applies to us all.

Remember that autonomy is associated with freedom. In Kant's view, freedom—as it applies to ethics—is the freedom *from* distractions that obscure from us the moral law. To be free is to be liberated from that which hides our obligations from us. To be free is to enjoy the certainty of knowing and intending to do what is right (Kant, 2010).

Consider the way that policies and laws compel action. Knowing that this is policy, you are now able to choose an action that fits within the boundaries that the policy sets. You are liberated—free—to choose an action within this boundary. You can make this choice with the confidence that you are on solid footing with respect to law and organizational policy. Administrative-level policies provide an abstract yet meaningful basis from which to choose how you will act. And yet, these regulations and policies are imposed on you by someone else—governments, employers, professional organizations. Even though these rules might make sense, the imposition of these rules from other people might seem like a restriction of your freedom.

However, what if there are rules on this administrative level that can serve as solid footing for your moral decision-making *and* such rules are given by you? That would be freedom. Such rules provide the freedom to know that you have firm direction to act rightly. And, since you are your own legislator, no one else is setting boundaries for you. Freedom to act, freedom from constraint. This, to Kant, is the moral law.

Kant saw that actions motivated by moral duty demonstrate respect to one's self as a moral legislator and to humanity as the universal subjects of duty. Just as Kant saw that actions motivated by moral duty demonstrate respect to one's self as a moral legislator and to humanity as the universal subjects of duty, so your active promotion of standards within the profession respects the profession itself.

The key to this moral law is the combination of you acting as your own legislator and rules that are reliable guides to right action. This means that, as your own legislator, you don't have the authority to just make up any rules that you wish. The rules that you set as duties have to pass a test—a test that will show that this rule really is worth accepting as a moral duty.

Kant offered the **categorical imperative** as this test to determine what our moral duties are. The term is meant to suggest that this test is seeking to identify commands that can be recognized and followed by moral agents (those are imperatives). These imperatives apply to us without exception (this is what *categorical* means).

The categorical imperative is to be used to test any potential principle (In Kantian terms, these are called *maxims*) to see if it should be seen as morally acceptable or—to the contrary—if we have a duty to never act on that principle. Any acceptable maxim needs to satisfy two conditions. First, a maxim that is a duty will be logically consistent and applicable in theory to all people. Second, it will be desirable for all people to follow. That is, we should be able to see that the world will

The **categorical imperative** is Immanuel Kant's test to determine what our moral duties are. It states: "Act always on a maxim that you can will to be a universal law."

be closer to the way it ought to be if everyone were to accept this rule as a duty(Kant, 2010).

The first condition of the categorical imperative tests the maxim logically to see if it can be applicable to all humanity. In other words, it has to be conceivable that this maxim could be held by all people as a duty. Any duty, then, must be one that, theoretically, can be followed by each and every person. This is a purely theoretical consideration. We cannot expect that everyone will follow any given maxim. But the categorical imperative is not inquiring into what people will do. It is looking to see what people should do.

If we find a conflict in which only some people can exercise a maxim, but not all, then the maxim cannot be a duty. Much immoral behavior consists of a contradiction in which someone wants to assert a difference between that person's duties and everyone else's. For instance: "I will steal but I don't want you to take my stuff."

The second condition of the categorical imperative is practical desirability. There is a gap between the world as it is and as it ought to be. A maxim that is a duty should be suited to help close that gap if everyone were to follow that maxim. Again, it doesn't matter how many people will actually follow that maxim. All that matters here is the abstract question of whether it is desirable for people to follow this maxim.

See what a **maxim** does. It is, first of all, a principle. As with any other principle, it sets boundaries and it categorizes. A maxim takes something like this form, *When I am in* this *kind of circumstance, I will act* this *way in order to bring this about*. Each this identifies a category: a category of circumstance, a category of action, and a category of the reason for doing the action. As with any principle, these categories are abstract. Even the *I* in a maxim is abstract. Not only does it refer to the moral agent who is considering this maxim, it also refers to any other rational human being who might be in this circumstance with the intention to bring about this result (Kant, 2010).

As an example, let's take this statement as a maxim to test: *If someone is in pain, I will do what I can to relieve that pain.* Can we imagine a world in which everyone will automatically respond to someone's pain by trying to offer some relief whenever they have the ability to offer that relief? In the abstract—which is all we need to consider at the administrative level—we can say *Yes*. Can we honestly expect everyone to be so responsive to pain in other people? No, but that's immaterial for this test. The categorical imperative is intended to determine what our moral duties are. That means that the test is looking toward how we ought to act, not toward how we can be expected to act. Talking about realistic expectations will belong to the strategic level.

This maxim also passes the second condition of the categorical imperative. Should we want people to alleviate pain when they are able to? If everyone were to act this way, would the world be better than it is? *Yes.*

Reliving pain in others passes the categorical imperative. This means that it is good—morally permissible—to act on this principle.

A **maxim** is a principle of action that connects an action with the reasons to perform it under certain circumstances.

This maxim identifies a category of circumstance—any time one is with someone in pain. It sets the category of a target result—any relief from that pain. Moreover, it identifies a category of action. In this case, the action is something of an abstract placeholder—whatever can be done. The categorical imperative asks you to imaginatively fit yourself in each of those categories, and also to imaginatively fit any and all rational human beings into those categories. Can we apply these categories to all people in this abstract way? (first condition); Should we want to? (second condition).

Therefore, this maxim passes the categorical imperative. This tells us that it is morally permissible to act on this maxim. Someone's in pain? You want to relieve that pain? Go ahead. You have the permission of humanity.

The categorical imperative is not simply a device to dole out permissions. At the administrative level, this is a tool to determine our boundaries. The example we've seen passes the categorical imperative and, therefore, is shown to be securely within the safe boundaries of moral permissibility. What happens when a maxim fails either of the two conditions of the categorical imperative?

The first condition of the categorical imperative tests to see if the maxim can be conceivably applied to all humanity. Kant saw this as a fundamental requirement of any moral duty—if it is a duty for one of us, it must be a duty for every one of us. Any maxim that cannot be accepted in theory as a plausible duty for everyone to follow fails at the most fundamental level. Such a miserable failure cannot be accepted as a principle for action at all. In Kant's terms, we have a *perfect duty* not to follow such a maxim. A perfect duty is a hard boundary. It is never acceptable to cross this line.

As an example, look back to the Niels Högel case given earlier. Högel's maxim—had he taken the time to deliberate in this way—might have been something like *I will place vulnerable people in greater mortal danger in order to try to save them.* You should be able to see that this is dramatically lacking in terms of practical desirability—and we haven't even explored that condition yet. This maxim is perhaps even worse from the standpoint of logical consistency. There is a contradiction here: We cannot expect all people to follow this at the same time. If we have all put each other in mortal danger, who is going to do the saving? We cannot possibly set a maxim like this as a duty for all people to follow. We, therefore, have a duty *never* to follow this maxim.

A maxim that meets the fundamental requirement of the second condition must show that adopting it by all humanity would bring us closer to the world as it ought to be. We'll state the obvious now: Failing this condition means that the maxim is not suited to make the world better than it is. You have, then, an *imperfect duty* not to follow this maxim. This means that you really shouldn't regard this maxim as morally acceptable, although it is understandable that you will act on it sometimes.

For example, Fernando is a radiologic technologist. His supervisor just informed him of an opportunity to attend a webinar at work that will count toward the continuing education (CE) requirements for his professional certification. Fernando recently had a periodic review at work with his supervisor, Patti, who noted that Fernando had several CE credits to complete for his renewal. While Fernando has another 6 months to complete the needed 6 credits, Patti suggests that he complete the requirement as soon as he can. Fernando understands the desirability of completing the credits, but his son is in the midst of his high school basketball season and he has been working extra shifts to pick up needed overtime pay. Fernando politely declines the invitation to the webinar. Fernando's maxim can be expressed: *When given the opportunity to enhance my knowledge and skills, I will decline that opportunity in order to save time.*

Fernando's maxim passes the first condition of the categorical imperative. We can envision a world in which people routinely decline opportunities to develop their skills in order to have more time for themselves. But would this bring us closer to the way the world ought to be? Would we want to live in such a world? It would be a stagnant world of undeveloped potential. Fernando's maxim fails the second condition of the categorical imperative. Fernando has an imperfect duty not to follow this maxim.

This does not mean that Fernando is being lazy. We've noted that he's working extra shifts, supporting his son's athletics, and he has satisfied most of the CE credits that he needs. All that we see here is that Fernando should not use this maxim routinely. We might even hope that Fernando feels a bit of regret at turning down this opportunity to advance his professional knowledge. Fernando's choice to turn down the opportunity for continuing education is not, by itself, morally desirable and he should feel no moral worth in turning down this opportunity. Even so, we should not view him harshly for this one instance of violating an imperfect duty.

On the other hand, imagine that Fernando were to attend the webinar. His maxim now might be: *When I find the opportunity for personal and professional improvement, I will make use of it.* From our analysis of the last example, we can see that this maxim will pass the categorical imperative. Having passed the categorical imperative, the maxim is morally acceptable. Any action taken by Fernando—or anyone else—on the basis of this maxim is permissible. Go ahead. Build those skills.

A maxim that passes the categorical imperative isn't necessarily a hard duty every time it might plausibly be put to use. We've already seen that it is understandable for Fernando to violate this maxim on some occasion. Consider also a maxim regarding giving money to worthy charities. Such a maxim might pass the categorical imperative, but it cannot reasonably require you to give all of your money to every charity. Acting on a successful maxim is a good thing to do. Where you really want to watch your duties, in the Kantian sense, is when they tell you what you shouldn't be doing.

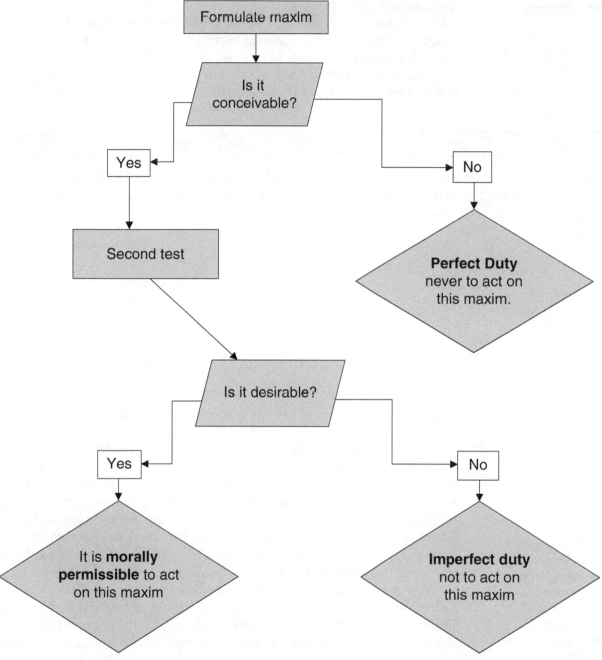

Figure 3.4 Categorical Imperative Flowchart

Beauchamp and Childress' four biomedical principles are also deontological. Each principle can be expressed as a Kantian maxim. For example, the principle of nonmaleficence could read: *When working with patients, I will not be a cause of harm to them.* You'll notice that no reason is given for not causing harm to patients. The desirability of not causing harm is self-evident. Don't cause harm to your patients. Just don't.

EXERCISE

Apply the categorical imperative to the nonmaleficence maxim just given. Does it pass? Next, express the principles of beneficence and justice as maxims. Use the categorical imperative to test each of them. What do you notice from this exercise?

The **humanity formulation of the categorical imperative** is a reformulated expression of Immanuel Kant's categorical imperative. It states: "Act in such a way that you treat humanity, yourself as well as any other person, never merely as a means to your own ends, but always at the same time as an end."

The categorical imperative clearly works with principles. Deontology is also concerned for rights. The categorical imperative can be taken as a device to reveal these to us as well. Högel's maxim, tested above, failed the categorical imperative because it cannot logically be applied to all people. Because it failed the test of logical consistency, we have an absolute duty never to act on this maxim. Put another way, each of us has a right not to be treated this way. Perfect duties imply rights. If I have a perfect duty not to do x to you, then you have a right not to have x done to you. If you have a right to autonomy, for instance, then everyone has an absolute duty to act with respect for your autonomy.

Respect for autonomy is the focus of another version of the categorical imperative. This is **the humanity formulation of the categorical imperative.** This formulation, fancy name and all, is meant to yield the same determinations of duty that we would find through the first expression of the categorical imperative. According to Kant, you respect your own autonomy as a moral legislator when you base your actions on moral duty. In the same way, acting on moral duty must also show respect for the autonomy of all other people (Kant, 2010).

To be treated as an end is to be treated as worthy of value. It is a goal, an important consideration. Anything that is treated merely as a means to some other end has no value of its own apart from the way it can be used to gain something else. If you force a group of people against their will to cook meals for you, then you are treating them merely as a means to your own end. On the other hand, you can go to a restaurant where a group of people will seat you, take your food order, cook the food, and serve it to you. Because they willfully accept this arrangement—and accept payment for the service—your action is acceptable. You are treating these workers at the restaurant as a means to your desired goal of a meal, but you are not treating them *merely* as a means to that goal.

The difference in the examples just given is consent. The restaurant workers solicit your business, are paid for their work, and agree to the entire arrangement. The emphasis of this formulation is on a perfect duty never to use people simply as an instrument to attain some other goal. Slavery, therefore, violates this perfect duty. Abuse of persons, including harassment, bullying, and discrimination will also violate this perfect duty. This is grounds for asserting that people have rights: There is a fundamental respect due to humanity, and people are entitled to this respect.

EXERCISE

Apply the humanity formulation of Immanuel Kant's categorical imperative to the informed consent process. In what way does this process respect people as rational beings?

Stressing the end of that last sentence, we need to caution against a leap that is sometimes taken: Immanuel Kant did not equate respect for autonomy with respect for someone's wishes. The way that other people want to be treated is not necessarily how they should be treated. Respect for autonomy, in the Kantian sense, means that we should treat people as they should want to be treated, or, rather, as they would want to be treated if they were autonomously thinking of moral duty. Properly, Kant's humanity formulation stresses respect for humanity. When any of us acts according to a maxim that passes the first formulation of the categorical imperative or treats one person as having the value that any member of humanity has, then humanity has been treated with respect.

Another important distinction to make is that the humanity formulation aims at respecting *humanity*. Remember that administrative-level assessment draws boundaries and categorizes. The humanity formulation addresses the category of humanity and accords respect to each human being because they are members of that set. Recognizing the value of humanity places boundaries with respect to how you can—and can't— treat human beings.

Now you can see why you were not asked to apply the categorical imperative to Beauchamp and Childress' principle of autonomy in the exercise above. Beauchamp and Childress oriented their attention to autonomy to respect for patients' choices. In their approach, respecting a patient's autonomy means providing information and allowing patients to make decisions. There is no expectation that patients must make rational decisions. There is respect for the decision maker even if the decision itself would violate the expectations of the categorical imperative (Beauchamp & Childress, 2013).

EXERCISE

Compare the notions of autonomy in Beauchamp and Childress' principle to Kant's use of the term.

Think about what happens when we do not act according to moral duty. In all, the picture of moral failure orients toward the basic expectation in Kantian ethics that we ought to act on the basis of moral duty. In the same way, we could argue that we ought to respect patient autonomy; and we ought to respect nonmaleficence, beneficence, and justice. These principles can seem so reasonable that we can wonder why we aren't always reliable in following them. Think back to the four vital intentions. Why, after all, are we inclined to cause harm? Why do we sometimes fail to do the good that we could? If these intentions are so fundamental, how are we able to fail to respect them?

Kant described three degrees of moral failure: frailty, impurity, and wickedness. We exhibit frailty when we identify what we ought to do, and desire to do it, but find that we are incapable of following duty. Such will be the case, for instance, when we face the hard task of trying to break a bad habit. We exhibit impurity when we act in a manner that is consistent with moral duty, but we also have other motivations to so act. Duty, in other words, is not the sole motivation. These two represent a lack of strength and, possibly, a lack of clarity. Wickedness represents what Kant called a perverse rejection of moral duty. The maxims of a wicked person are not those that can conceivably be willed to be followed by all; they only serve the perceived interests of the individual (Kant, 1960).

EXERCISE

Apply the categorical imperative to the four vital intentions earlier in the chapter. Express each intention as a maxim and test it. What added perspective does this exercise provide into our interest in promoting good and avoiding harm?

THEORY AND DECISION-MAKING AIDS

Administrative-level ethical assessment takes the larger view.

When you examine a policy or regulation, examine it at the level on which it applies. In other words, don't just look at what it means for you, right now, to act on this principle. At this close range, you might miss the intent of the policy. Instead, take a few steps back and look for the value in the policy.

Ethical assessment aims at modulating our moral reactions, helping us to arrive at better perspectives and better actions than we would otherwise have by relying on our moral reactions alone. As noted in Chapter 1, our moral reactions can be flawed. Now, seeing the administrative level of assessment in some detail, we can recognize a little more of where our moral reactions can leave something to be desired. Morality is a mix of perception of harm, emotional response, conceptual categorization, and motivation to act. All of these can wrap together with an intention to do good. That intention is a general wish. We want good things to happen and we want to be happy and safe. But that general intention isn't always matched by more specific intentions in the moment that are conducive to actually positioning us to bring about the good we desire.

We sometimes live under the myth that we are of one mind all or most of the time. Upon reflection, we find that we are minds of many angles. What we think, feel, and desire can compete instead of partner. We can act despite our emotions. We can act against our better motivations. Ethical assessment seeks to add another angle to the collage— one of executive control that seeks to clarify our perceptions, refine our cognition, deliberate upon our motivations, and set upon a course of action that we can defend as the best we could do.

ASSESSMENT FROM THE ADMINISTRATIVE LEVEL

Ethical skills at the administrative level involve setting boundaries. This is a large-scale form of putting things in perspective. When you approach a moral issue, begin by assessing the issue from the standpoint of the principles autonomy, nonmaleficence, beneficence, and justice. What stands out as you apply each one? Do you see any conflicts between these principles? If so, note these for further examination. Consider how you will prioritize these.

Examine the issue through application of Kant's categorical imperative: If a principle is being invoked, can it theoretically apply to everyone? (Kant's first condition) Does this policy or principle appear directed toward bringing the world (the health-care system, this hospital) closer to the way it ought to be? Using the humanity formulation of the categorical imperative, consider if anyone is being used merely as a means to further someone else's goals.

These efforts will help position you to test a policy or principle and find its value. On the administrative level, we are looking for value in the abstract. The general intention is to do good matched with a reasonable way of addressing good for all and an idea of how this good should look in the world.

STRATEGIC LEVEL

The strategic level of ethical assessment involves the analysis of plans of action according to the likelihood that they will yield harm or benefit. This is the level at which determinations are made about what course of action to take. Options will be considered here. Potential outcomes of those options are weighed.

At the strategic level, we modulate perceptions as we check to determine that we have detail that is accurate and reasonably complete. From this detail, we are able to engage a practical assessment of goals that we might seek to bring about and options to help bring about those goals. The match of goal and option that stands to bring about the best consequences is the right one to select and act upon.

Administrative-level assessment provides some guidelines for strategic assessment. The administrative level draws boundaries and sets categories. These efforts establish a certain efficiency in our moral decision-making. This is necessary as a way to manage time constraints. But sometimes we face situations that are not neatly addressed by the principles and policies at our disposal. Sometimes, there is controversy about what to do. Sometimes people have different perspectives and different value systems that prevent them from seeing eye to eye on a moral matter. In these cases, our efficient decision-making approaches run into a snag. We, therefore, need the ability to be flexible enough to review just how the principles should apply.

Flexibility can also demand that we look outside our given principles in order to arrive at a fresh perspective and the best decision. Often—particularly in cases where there is moral controversy—plausible courses of action will produce some good and some harm. In such a case, there isn't a clear option where we can benefit the patient without causing any harm at all. Beneficence and nonmaleficence don't provide a means to determine how much good we cause and how much harm we might cause. We already know that we don't want to cause harm and that we want to provide benefit. The challenge is in knowing how to make this happen.

A flexible theory will be able to address the particulars of a situation and the options available to us. We can use this approach to help compare different options as we try to weigh their relative advantages and disadvantages and try to decide which option is the better choice.

At the administrative level, we work with broad conceptualizations. Our assessment at that level occurs from considerable distance, at which vantage point finer distinctions blur. We close this distance for strategic-level assessment. Colors are nuanced, edges and angles are defined. Strategic-level assessment has to respond to situational differences as details emerge and take on importance.

Details are vitally important. The information gained determines the best course of action to take. Without adequate attention to detail, we are prone to misinformed action. The strategic level is rather like the ethical version of a head-to-toe assessment. As clinical nursing assessments have a positive impact on patient outcomes upon entering, and being discharged from, hospitals, so strategic-level assessment is essential to effective and practical action.

At the same time, there are a lot of details and you only have so much time. Above, it was stated that we seek detail that is accurate and *reasonably complete*. Kind of vague, isn't it? We can't hold the expectation that you know everything there is to know about a situation—that's almost certainly impossible. But we do hold the expectation that you put good effort into identifying what really needs to be known. The confounding factor is time. If all you had was one patient, a head-to-toe assessment could take hours. You could gather exhaustive detail and then go back over it to sort out what's important to know and what isn't. But, in practice, how much time do you have for this assessment? 20 minutes? 15? 10? Again, this is all vague. And it is shaped by context and situation. In some situations, you have impossible demands on your time. In some situations, a few details about a patient will especially stand out as very important. How do you know whether to act on such details right away or to keep going with the assessment lest you overlook something else that is important but less obvious?

Strategic-level thinking is highly situational and often complicated. The situation is shaped by a unique and variable set of details that strongly impact upon the decision to be made. This is the same with clinical and ethical assessments. In this situation, the time available to gather information will vary. You are not a distant observer, watching events unfold that do not involve you. Being in position to make this level of ethical assessment means that something is happening now that needs your attention. You might have enough time to do a thorough investigation and arrive at a thoughtful decision. Or, you might have to think fast because events are moving and won't slow down for you.

And there are so many details in any given situation. Not all of those details will be ethically relevant. For the most part, you are already practiced in sorting this out. We naturally build a perception of the world in which we sort out what is important/noticeable from what is not to be noticed. Again, executive control can be part of this process. Wondering if you know enough or if you are seeing relevant details clearly is good opening strategy.

In principle, each of the four vital intentions has merit. In practice, conflicts among these intentions can arise. We all know that efforts to address suffering may create other forms of suffering, such as pain from a needle injection, side effects from medication, or the stress involved in waiting for test results. Strategic level thinking, therefore, frequently requires weighing of benefits versus harms.

ALREADY IN PRACTICE

There is clear overlap between the administrative and the strategic levels. The rules crafted as guides for behavior are shaped by an interest in what we actually do and the outcomes that stream from those actions. In other words, we craft administrative guidelines because we are moral agents whose actions matter in the world. Notions of principles, rights and virtues all aim in some way toward promoting effective agency in the world.

Policies and procedures are communication tools used to achieve specific outcomes. The effect of crafting procedures from the guidance of policies is to streamline the decision-making process and encourage predictability and reliability in our actions. While there is high variability in the details of any specific situation, there might be enough essential details that we can offer a standard process to address them. Protocols are standardized methods tailored to consistently produce a specific outcome.

Decision-making processes that are regulated often belong to situations that present common details that have special moral weight. Typically, these will be situations in which some significant harm is at stake. Procedures can guide actions for the purpose of protecting safety or for the purpose of facilitating some good and necessary outcome.

Because of the importance assigned to the outcomes of certain procedures, compliance can be expected. *Compliance* is obedience to expectations for behavior that are set by others. We will be able to see that compliance can be an area of concern in the strategic level—such as a compliance with a nursing protocol, or a patient's compliance with medication orders. At the administrative level, compliance is the demonstration of adherence to rules.

Compliance can be tracked and measured in an effort to ensure orderly conduct. The individual meets the expectations for following the procedure or protocol. Many aspects are involved in compliance. These professional obligations include integrity and the principles of biomedical ethics.

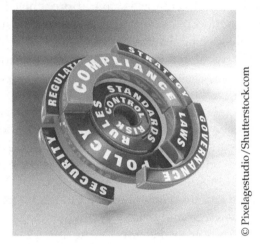

Figure 3.5

Not all actions can be guided by protocols. For issues that cannot be guided by protocols—and to review the effectiveness of existing protocols—we are left to figure out how to make decisions. What follows next is an exploration of utilitarianism—one of the best-known theoretical approaches to strategic decision-making.

NORMATIVE THEORY

Consequentialist theories ask us to avoid causing harm and to produce benefit. These approaches direct us to analyze available courses of action in order to determine which option stands to produce the optimum outcome. In a consequentialist outlook, an action gains moral value as it produces good outcomes.

In consequentialist ethics, actions become right or wrong depending on their outcomes. The fundamental ethical goal in strategic-level assessment is to bring about practical benefit. Consequentialist theories focus on this goal and use the results of our actions as criteria for determining their moral worth. This sounds direct, but the task is complicated.

Actions are undertaken in specific situations by specific people. Administrative-level abstraction isn't available. To evaluate an action, we have to do so within the context in which it will take place. It is tempting to judge actions in hindsight. This is useful for the purposes of reassessing our choices, but the intent of strategic-level decision-making is to determine what to do. It always points toward the future. Actions have to be judged on the basis of the outcomes that we can anticipate from them. For these reasons, consequentialist theories have to emphasize careful attention to detail. In order to understand the context in which action will take place, there must be careful evidence gathering. In order to properly assess the outcomes that we can anticipate from an action, we must have sound and complete information about this sort of action and its likely results.

Because consequentialist theories have approaches that are designed to weigh both production of benefit and avoidance of harm, they have more *flexibility*. Consider again the strength with which deontological theories can tell us what not to do compared to telling us what we ought to do.

The capacity to weigh benefit against harm provides a means to declare an obligation where deontology cannot. In the case of giving to those in need, a consequentialist will look at the specifics of a given situation. What good can be offered? What harm can be avoided? Might any harm be created? How do the benefits and harms of this situation compare to other options that are available to you? In the course of this analysis, a judgment can be reached about whether a particular option can be seen as worthwhile and even as obligatory.

Return to the example of Fernando and his CE credits. The categorical imperative showed that Fernando has an imperfect duty not to give up the opportunity for professional development. But we saw that Fernando had reasons for doing so. In a consequentialist evaluation, those benefits of working overtime and supporting his son's athletics might outweigh the benefit he would receive from the webinar.

How is Fernando to make a decision about whether or not to register for this webinar? **Consequentialism** is a general outlook that points Fernando in the direction of making his choice by measuring possible outcomes. But consequentialism itself offers no guidance for doing this. For guidance, we turn to utilitarianism, a version of consequentialism.

THEORY AND DECISION-MAKING AIDS

Utilitarian theories advocate a method through which you weigh the beneficial and harmful consequences at stake for a given course of action and weigh them to determine the relative moral worth of pursuing this action. The option that stands to produce the greatest surplus of benefit over harm is the best intervention to pursue.

The core idea of **utilitarianism** is to produce the greatest amount of good that we can. We can express the main utilitarian principle this way: *The right action is the option that produces the greatest balance of outcomes for the community* (Bentham, 1996; Mill, 1998).

Consequentialism is a style of normative ethics that makes determinations about right or wrong action according to the outcomes produced by those actions.

Utilitarianism is a normative ethical theory that advocates a decision-making method that promotes acting to produce the best overall consequences for the greatest number of people.

Several points need to be kept in mind. First, the utilitarian is looking for the greatest surplus of benefit over harm. An act that produces moderate benefit and only a small amount of harm is preferable to an act that produces extensive benefit along with slightly less (but still extensive extensive) harm.

EXERCISE

As a good utilitarian, Fernando needs some way to assess the relative amount of benefit and harm at stake in the options available to him. What are his options? What can you say about the balance of benefit and harm for each option?

Second, utilitarianism is at its best when it evaluates options. It is nice to know that an action you plan to undertake promises to produce more benefit than harm. It is another thing to realize that this action has greater promise in this regard than any other option that is available to you. Consider a treatment decision for a patient. Aggressive treatment that presents extensive risk of adverse effects will only be recommended if there are no better options to bring about desired health outcomes. A *better* option, in other words, would be one that can deliver the same outcomes but do so with less risk of harm and suffering to the patient.

EXERCISE

Odilia is worried about her daughter, Natalie. Natalie is 12. She complains of chills and body aches. Odilia believes that Natalie has the flu. What worries her is Natalie's temperature, 39.1C. Odilia thinks that the flu can just pass after a week or so, but the fever has her concerned. She wonders if she should take Natalie in to the Emergency Department. What are Odilia's options? From a utilitarian standpoint, which option is the best?

Third, your evaluation of options must take account of outcomes that you can reasonably anticipate. Most of all, this means that you should not just evaluate an action on the assumption that everything will work out as you plan. You know that our best intentions do not always come to fruition. Before you act, think carefully about what might happen. Think of giving a medication that has known side effects. It is not enough to give the medication and expect everything to work as intended. You need to be prepared for the possibility that an adverse reaction might occur. In the same way, your evaluation of options under a utilitarian approach should account for adverse events that you can reasonably anticipate.

Fourth, your evaluation must account for the impact of your action on all individuals who stand to be affected. As used above, the term *community* refers to all such individuals. Standing on an administrative-level notion of moral equality, utilitarianism asserts that each person has the same moral worth as any other person.

Part of the intent of this focus on community is to encourage objective assessment untainted by bias against certain persons. No one person is to count any more or less than any other. Keep this in mind as you consider that utilitarianism, as a strategic-level decision-making method, is intended for use in making hard decisions in which some people benefit while others receive harm. Consider a trauma situation in which multiple casualties are triaged. Under normal triage conditions (see Chapter 9 for complications), critical cases will be taken first, and minor cases will receive treatment last. The critical cases are given priority. This is not done so because they count more, but because giving priority to them is the most effective way to bring about good outcomes for all individuals involved.

Finally, there is a need for nuance as you investigate possible outcomes. Any action can lead to multiple consequences. Some of these consequences will arise quickly while others will unfold at a later time. Some consequences will be long-lasting while others will quickly fade away. Some consequences will bring both benefit and harm. Some will bring benefit that later turns to harm. It is tempting to reduce utilitarianism to a swift exercise in counting who benefits and who doesn't. Sometimes this approach might work. Often, we need to be more attentive to the details. What is really at stake? What can we really expect as we consider a particular action, and how does it compare to alternatives?

There is work in utilitarianism. The theory is asking you to think long and hard about what you do. An action isn't recommended just because you think you can achieve something worthwhile through it. The method is designed to compel you to think of who your action will impact and how. You need to think carefully about what kind of impact your action might have. Moreover, you need to think of alternatives. Your action can have wide-reaching effect. Make the most of it that you can.

ETHICAL COMPETENCY AT THE STRATEGIC LEVEL

Ethical skills at the strategic level involve identifying and weighing options. Begin with an assessment of the different courses of action that might be pursued. If there is a conflict of opinion between people, identify the courses of action they advocate. Are there other options aside from the ones they support?

Engage a utilitarian analysis to sort out what is at stake for each option. Carefully gather facts about the situation. What is at stake? Who stands to be affected?

Carefully identify the options available in this situation. For each option assess all attending beneficial and harmful outcomes that can be reasonably anticipated. Weigh these potential consequences for each option. Is there greater promise of benefit than risk of harm? If so, how great is the difference? Of the available options, which one promises the greatest balance of benefit over harm for all individuals involved?

Discuss this assessment with your colleagues and, if appropriate, with the patient or the patient's family. Is it possible to arrive at a consensus?

INTERPERSONAL LEVEL

Compassion is the one thing you don't need doctor's orders for.

The interpersonal level is found in that moment when one person directly interacts with another. In this encounter, a moral agent recognizes the other as a person of moral value. What the moral agent does matters to this other person. (Of course, in many encounters, both people are moral agents.) Here, there is witness to suffering and personal opportunity to alleviate suffering and to nurture conditions for good.

The administrative level provides guidelines and boundaries. The strategic level sets a plan of action. Once the action is determined, there remains the matter of the actual delivery. This is the interpersonal level. This is the level of participation.

Compassion is not uniformly understood or defined. Differences in culture, individual perspective and language have produced wide-ranging treatments of compassion among different theoretical and scientific efforts to explore the phenomenon (Gilbert, 2017). Some sources begin with an assumption that compassion is a feeling, an affective state. Such an assumption will have trouble distinguishing compassion from empathy. It was shown in Chapter 1 that empathy plays some role in our moral reactions. Just as Chapter 1 demonstrated ethical thinking as different from having a moral reaction, so it will be maintained here that compassion is different from empathy. Compassion, then, will not be treated as primarily a feeling or affective state. Compassion is described here as a sort of **willingness**—a motivational state. With willingness, there needs to be awareness.

Compassion is the willingness to be responsive to another person who suffers and to establish an interpersonal connection that affirms the importance and worth of that person.

Willingness is an attitude in which one opens to the suffering and personhood of another.

Awareness and willingness are the two pillars on which compassion stands. The process of compassion involves a reflexive relationship between awareness and willingness, complemented by responses. There can be degrees of willingness and awareness. They can fuel each other. Having willingness can inspire one to become aware. Being aware can inspire more motivation to respond to the suffering of another. Awareness includes critical thinking and the effort to gather detail. The more you know, the better you are able to respond. In the immediate face of suffering, or threat of suffering, we have three main options: fight, flight or freeze. Or, to put these in another way: act, escape, or pause.

A literal reading of compassion yields *suffering with*. This etymological origin, by itself, doesn't suggest a difference from sympathy or empathy. For the purposes of this text, and to present a view that is consistent with some trends in research, the terms are further developed here.

Sympathy is recognizing that another person is capable of suffering. (Anticipating that someone could be harmed even though they don't see it coming.) This can also be abstract, such as recognizing that people have rights (Keen, 2006).

Consider that the interpersonal level of ethical assessment entails close proximity to someone who suffers. For our purposes, then, compassion can be seen as being with someone who suffers, aware of this suffering, and willing to be in that proximity and responsive to the needs of the one who suffers. Empathy means suffering in response to the observation of someone else's suffering. The person who feels empathy is motivated to address the suffering that he or she feels. The person who is compassionate is motivated to address the suffering of the other person.

Empathy can manifest in different forms. As discussed in Chapter 1, empathy is an emotional response in which the suffering of someone else is mirrored as a distress that you feel. Empathy manifests in different ways. Emotional contagion is the experience in which you mirror someone else's distress but feel that pain as if it were your own. In a nursery, for example, all it takes is for one infant to cry. That wailing little voice will be joined by other wails throughout the nursery. The infants are not crying because they are concerned for the welfare of the first infant to cry. They are responding to their own distress—distress that was brought on by mirroring the distress of the first child (Buchanan, Bagley, Stansfield, & Preston, 2012; Keen, 2006; Martin et al., 2015).

We might say that the truer form of empathy arises when you are aware that your distress is a response to the suffering you witness in someone else. We are remarkably adept at placing an emotional investment in others. We are capable of feeling empathy for people who are personally connected with us because we know them or because we witness their suffering. We can also feel empathy for pets and other nonhuman animals. We even can feel empathy for characters that we know to be fictional. This latter kind of "storied empathy" (Commons & Wolfsont, 2002; Gruen, 2009) is made possible in part by an act of imagination. You are removed from the characters and know that there is no action you can take on their behalf. Your emotional stress you feel as the plot moves will resolve as the story comes to an end. Emotional contagion and storied empathy do not inspire agency.

But empathy motivates you to act. Agential actions from empathy arise when you feel the suffering of another, recognize that you are suffering in response to this person's suffering, and feel the added motivation to act to address the suffering that you feel. However, your source of information—that which you take to be an indicator of what the other person feels and needs—is *your own suffering*. There is an inherent bias in empathy. You act on the basis of your experience, transposing that to the other person whom you make the target of your caring action. Since the other person might not feel as you do, your caring action might be misguided and poorly received.

Empathy can also be a poor ethical guide. The main motivation in empathy is to put a stop to the suffering that you feel—even if this is not the intention you consciously express or recognize. Overwhelmed by this suffering, you might find that you respond with a fight/flight/ or flee reaction that prevents you from cognitively assessing the problem and determining an appropriate course of action to address it. Empathy can be inconsistent or irrational in the actions it motivates. Your empathy for people you identify with (your in-group) can bias you against the interests of people who are not in your in-group. Empathy can impede compassion (Decety & Cowell, 2015; Prinz, 2011).

When someone says, *If it were my mother, I would…* they are engaging agential empathy, not compassion. Being compassionate means refraining from interjecting your own feelings. Relying on the suffering you feel to offer guidance to your patient is empathetic, but it may also be paternalistic, presumptuous, and—worse—a poor fit for what the patient needs. Compassionate care helps patients gain perspective, frame decisions, and identify and express their needs.

This is not to say that empathy is regrettable, nor that we should feel it. Empathy can indeed be valuable in establishing connections between people, and it can serve as a motivation to ethical action. The point to be acknowledged at this point is that empathy—an instinctive moral feeling—is insufficient by itself as a moral guide. Further, empathy is a stress response; it produces suffering of its own (Loggia, Mogil, & Catherine, 2008). We can do better on the interpersonal level. Particularly, we can draw on our capacity to witness others in their suffering, to be open to paying attention to them, to have the willingness to attend to their needs, and to reach out to aid them with a critical awareness of what they need. This is compassion (Bloom, 2016).

Compassion entails some cognitive and interpersonal effort to assess the situation. Gather facts, pay attention to the other person, connect with the other person, think of possible courses of action, determine which course of action is the best among the options available to you.

Compassion is directed toward the other person. Instead of a reactive response to the suffering you feel, compassion entails the capacity to pay attention to the other person. In that awareness, you develop a critical understanding of what the other person needs. Your willingness is, first, to be present with this person and, second, to do what you can to be responsive to that person's needs.

Empathy manifests as a desire to fix. Not all suffering can be fixed. Facing this recognition, an empathetic person can panic and flee or freeze in uncertainty. Compassion is marked with the willingness to pay attention to the person who suffers. In this compassionate willingness, you may be aware that you cannot fix this person's suffering, but you are also aware that your compassionate attention establishes an important interpersonal connection between the two of you.

We have no unit of measuring compassion. It is not a strategic outcome. Compassion can't be planned, but it can be cultivated. Compassion is a form of giving. It is an association in which both parties reach out. One reaches out for help. The one with compassion reaches out to help. The compassionate one gives. If nothing else, you compassionately give of yourself to your patient (Sinclair et al., 2016; van der Cingel, 2011).

Compassion is different from altruism. Altruism entails putting other people ahead of you. Altruism can also be defined as a sort of willingness: specifically, a willingness to place others ahead of yourself. We all do this occasionally. Altruism, however, is a belief that one ought to largely subsume the self to the good of others. In terms of giving; we might see this as a giving away of what you have and of who you are. There can be moments where self-sacrifice is necessary and heroic. As a prevailing attitude, however, it saps your resources. This is the avenue to stress or burnout.

Compassion includes self-compassion. Compassionate giving isn't for the sake of giving yourself away. In giving of yourself compassionately to someone else, you also give to yourself. There is a sense of worth in your act and a sense of interpersonal connection with the one to whom you connect interpersonally. In compassionate action, you manage yourself so that you can attend to the other person.

EXERCISE

You walk into a patient's room to find that the patient is nauseated and vomiting. What is compassionate action in this case? How might empathy get in the way of effective action on the patient's behalf?

CARE AND COMPASSION

The administrative and strategic levels can help you gain perspective and move beyond the hold of your empathetic suffering. Think of the levels of ethical assessment in terms of distance.

At the farthest distance you have a broad perspective from which you can see many people. They are so distant from you that you do not feel personally connected with any single person. The distance is so far removed that individual characteristics cannot be made out. You can tell that you are looking at people, but you can't make out gender, race, ethnicity, or other distinguishing features. You only see humanity. You can have a *sympathetic* concern for all of these people, but you can't develop a close connection for any one of them. That is, you recognize that all of these people matter as individuals even though none of them matter to you more than the rest. This is the view from the administrative level.

In the middle distance, you are close enough to see and interact with people. Differences are apparent. You can see that no two people are alike. You also recognize that these people face different challenges and circumstances. You stand far enough removed, however, that you are able to take a larger view of their situations and offer advice. This is the view from the strategic level.

Both of these distances involve a way of *caring about* people. You care about someone who is close to you by placing your wish that this person not suffer. You care about people who are remote for you by holding the abstract wish that no one suffer.

At the interpersonal level, you are immediately present with another person. You sit with someone who suffers. You reach out to help this person and this person reaches out for your help.

Compassion is caring for. *Caring for* entails committing your efforts to address someone's best interests. Particularly, to reduce their suffering and to prevent them from coming to harm. Even if you only care about someone in an abstract, sympathetic way, it is still possible to care for them. It is possible to care for someone even if you do not care about someone because this person has threatened to cause you harm or because this person seems otherwise heinous to you.

This means that you can offer compassionate care even if you do not feel a close empathetic connection to someone. Part of the concern about empathy as a moral guide is that we don't feel empathy consistently for everyone. People who do not fit into our in-groups may not appeal to us as objects of empathy. We might have a hard time mustering empathy for those who displease us or threaten us (Prinz, 2011). Compassion, however, aligns with critical thinking and conscious efforts to modulate intuitive reactions. While empathy can inspire compassion in us, compassionate care can be also directed toward those who do not appear to us to be objects of empathy.

It is possible to offer compassionate care and carry out your professional expectations to all of your patients. Compassion rests in willingness and awareness. It involves critical thinking. It requires the humility to sit with someone in their suffering. There is no requirement that you establish an emotional attachment to the one who reaches out for your help. What they need is your compassionate attention.

NARRATIVE

We are meaning-seeking beings. We have a drive to make sense of who we are and with whom we belong. We seek significance in what we can do and in who we can be. We wrap our moral agency into narratives about the influence we can have on the world and on other people who matter to us. Attending to narrative is an important way to enhance and cultivate compassion (Charon, 2008).

Narrative refers to an effort by people to identify meaning in their lives. This is done through the telling, and receiving, of a story of who that person is and with whom that person belongs.

Narrative is a form of critical thinking. We tell stories about our lives. There is a basic need in each of us to have someone listen to us and say, "What is happening to you matters because it is happening to you."

While some work in the study of narrative focuses on the interest in crafting a coherent story, it is meaning that is the real interest that drives our narrative efforts. The experience of illness provides key insight. Arthur W. Frank identifies three types of narrative used to describe illness experience. The *restitution narrative* is the story we all want to tell: a tale of temporary suffering that ends with the restoration of health and a return to one's normal life. The *quest narrative* is a more heroic tale, in which the protagonist has been transformed through illness and recovery, and now has a mission. The *chaos narrative*—listed second by Frank—is told in the midst of illness. This narrative is told from the perspective of one whose life is disrupted. The story is hard to tell and harder to hear (Frank, 2013).

In a chaos narrative the interest is in crafting a narrative of meaning. Coherence takes a back seat. We know that people often weave elements into their narratives that they recognize as untrue (Frankfurt, 2010). But the narratives—and their identities—become more interesting this way.

Chaos narratives cannot be told in linear fashion. The purpose for telling them is not to put things in order but to struggle for meaning. The chaos narrative is written in despair. The possibility of hope for the future is severely challenged. The narrative represents both a lament at the loss of meaning and a desperate attempt to struggle for meaning. A chaos narrative cannot be told coherently. The lack of the possibility of coherence is the reason why the chaos narrative needs to be told. It is a struggle for meaning, not a struggle for coherence (Frank, 2013).

The importance of narrative highlights the need for attention to the interpersonal level of ethics. A narrative isn't simply told. It is co-created through the work of a narrator and an attentive audience. In telling a story, the narrator looks for meaning. Meaning is not solely centered on the individual but locates the individual in a social world to which the individual belongs. The narrative has to gain meaning through its acceptance by an audience. Your story of who you are takes on meaning as others hear it and respond to it. In their response, there is some acknowledgment that your story matters. The most important factor of the audience's response is the act of attentive listening. In paying attention, the audience affirms the significance of the narrative. By paying attention to the narrative, the narrative is shown to be worth listening to. The narrator is worth being heard.

The interpersonal aspect of ethical assessment is a way of seeing the person you are facing. The ideal is to create an interpersonal connection that is fulfilling to both you and the person you face. Some refer to this ideal as **authentic presence** (Watson, 2008).

To be present authentically is to pay profound attention to the other person. There are no rules or protocols here. There is no posture that needs to be adopted and no requirement for eye contact. Posture and comportment flow appropriately if one thing is kept in mind: Be willing to hear what this person has to say. Presence is profound if you look to the other person as significant, as if that person has greater value to you right now than anything else.

Authentic presence is compassionate attention to another person, affirming the others person's status as someone who matters.

Thich Nhat Hanh offers a model for authentic presence in the Bodhisattva, Ksitigarbha (also known as Jizo). An embodiment of compassion, Ksitigarbha refuses to abandon those who suffer. In the depths—the chaos, the hell—of your suffering, Ksitigarbha remains with you. He sits with you and listens (Thich Nhat Hanh, 1998). There is no judgment. There is no advice. There is presence. There is the gift of attention and the unqualified demonstration that you matter, your suffering matters. You have a narrative that is worthy of attention. And so, you, in the depth of your misery, still matter. You have not lost that. There is hope because there is still a connection that you can have with one who listens to you (Hall, 2005).

The image of Ksitigarbha depicts someone who walks into the dark, into a prison cell, at a hospital bed, into a corner of hell to sit with someone in pain. Authentic presence places you with someone in the midst of their suffering. As you open to this person's narrative, you also open yourself to that person's pain. There is humility and vulnerability in the act of compassion. The vow of authentic presence, *I will listen to you because you matter,* is a vow of willingness. It can be easier on us to hold people at a distance—their pain remains with them. Compassion entails the willingness to draw close and to be open to empathy and the mirrored suffering that can follow. Through compassionate connection it is possible to overcome that suffering and transform the experience you share with the one who suffers (Angel & Vatne, 2017).

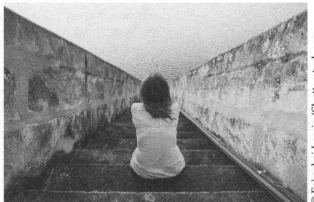

Figure 3.6

To further show the importance of narrative, consider the case of perhaps the most profoundly anonymous patient in medical history: Henrietta Lacks. She died of cervical cancer on October 4, 1951. While under treatment, cell samples from her tumor were taken and cultured. Remarkably, the cell line proved to be immortal, resisting apoptosis and reproducing indefinitely under the right laboratory conditions. Lacks never consented to experiments on her tissue. Her identity was distanced from the cells, which were named *HeLa* (Skloot, 2010).

This cell line has been among the most significant of developments in medical science. Yet, the woman that the cells came from remained obscured from the scientists who researched them and from the patients who derived benefit from some of that research.

After Lacks died, the lab assistant who cultured the HeLa cells was directed to attend the autopsy in order to gather more tissue samples. To this point, the assistant had been as unaware of the person as researchers who experimented with the cells. The assistant took on a new view when she gazed at Henrietta Lacks' feet and noticed her nail polish. "I thought, *Oh jeez, she's a real person.* I started imagining her sitting in the bathroom painting those toenails, and it hit me for the first time that those cells we've been working with . . . came from a live woman."[1]

Henrietta Lacks was a real person. Like all of us, she lived a life in search of meaning. That search speaks. In authentic presence, we hear this voice. We can hear it in small moments—the context of painting your nails or of taking tissue samples. Henrietta Lacks didn't paint her nails in order to put meaning to her life, of course. She did this simply as part of the course of her life. But that course is where the significance needs to be found. In her normal life, just as she was, Henrietta Lacks mattered.

You will see patients who are desperate to convey this. Illness takes them out of their normal lives. In their normal routines, it never occurred to them that they might not be significant. They had narratives that were readily accepted by others. They belonged. Now, the routine is gone but they remain. They sometimes wonder if their significance stayed with them or if that went along with everything else they lost. Read a cancer memoir. Notice how often people affirm the refrain, *I am here* (Broyard, 1993; Conway, 2007; Host, 2011; Fies, 2008; Lorde, 2006; Middlebrook, 1998; Radner, 2009).

ETHICAL COMPETENCY AT THE INTERPERSONAL LEVEL

Ethical skills at the interpersonal level involve seeing the person.

Begin by identifying the person you are with now. Who is this person? Pay attention. What can you learn from the narrative this

---

[1] Quoted in Skloot, pp. 90–91. Emphasis is the author's.

person offers? What does this person need from you now? How can you help?

Identify the person who has the greatest vulnerability in this situation. Who is this person? Pay attention. What can you learn from the narrative this person offers? What does this person need from you now? How can you help?

Identify the person who has the most pressing need of you. Who is this person? Pay attention. What can you learn from the narrative this person offers? What does this person need from you now? How can you help?

It is possible that the same person will be identified in these three questions. If these questions identify two or more people, consider where you are needed most.

Who else is involved in this situation. What recognition do they need from you? Is there a way to help them?

What about you? What does this situation mean to you? How do you see yourself?

PUTTING IT ALL TOGETHER

The imagery of each of these levels of assessment as a vantage point is essential to the intended use of this model of assessment. The point is to expand your moral vision. Recall the account of moral feelings in Chapter 1: Your perception of an event arises with a cognitive labeling and a motivation. In other words, your intuitive moral beliefs correlate strongly with the way in which you perceive an event or issue. But, this perspective is limited and includes misperceptions that lead to off-base judgments. While your moral feelings are often reliable guides to good behavior, they are prone to flaws that can lead to embarrassing situations, conflicts, and poor decisions. You can do better. The place to start is to expand your perspective.

It's important to remember that moral issues are not purely academic issues. While we use hypothetical or historical case studies and questions in a text like this, the real test of ethical competency is in your life. The ethical arena is the living, social world around you now. This means that any moral issue you face is going to involve other people. These other people will also approach this issue through their own perspectives, which will differ from yours in some way. Sometimes, different perspectives will clash, adding a level of conflict to the moral issue. Other times, there will be some coherence among different perspectives, yet subtle differences will exist that can lend differing insight to the problem at hand. Moreover, of course, many issues will contain a mix of clashing and compatible perspectives. Life is complex, after all.

ETHICAL COMPETENCY AND THE ART OF ASSESSMENT

Ethics is an activity. It is a skill to be used to clarify situations of moral significance and to determine how we should act. Ethical competency is the ability to reliably exercise ethical skills. Ethical competency won't make you a moral saint, but it can have noticeable benefits in helping you to set priorities, clarify your tasks, and to avoid and resolve conflicts.

We might think of ethical skills as "soft skills." Hard skills are those that can be described in a step-by-step fashion and measured according to some sort of analytic process. You can learn to place an IV. You can learn proper charting procedures. You can learn the skills for donning and removing PPE. Communication skills, listening skills, and compassion are softer. We are reasonably good at knowing when people are very good or very bad at listening, but it can be hard to explain exactly how we know this. Moreover, when someone is bad at listening, it can be hard to point out exactly what this person is doing poorly.

Ethical skills involve communication, listening, and compassion. They involve some capacity to balance your emotions, and to reflect before reacting. Ethical skills involve critical thinking and perspective-building. As a set of soft skills, a step-by-step method for ethical conduct can't be offered. However, it is possible to offer a model to help in the effort to build perspective and encourage you in the use of the other necessary skills. To help address a moral issue, develop the skills to view the situation through the administrative, strategic and interpersonal levels.

ETHICAL ASSESSMENT MODEL

To facilitate your assessment of a moral situation, it can be useful to use the following Ethical Assessment Model:

SITUATION
- What is happening now?
- What are the facts?
- What policies, procedures, or orders apply?
- Who is suffering now and in what way? Is anyone at risk of harm, and in what way?
- What is the conflict?
- What background is relevant to understanding the situation?

BACKGROUND/PEOPLE
- Who is involved?
- What are the expectations and ideas of the people in this situation?

- What background is relevant to understanding the people in this situation?
- What are your initial reactions and intuitions about this situation?

LEVELS OF ASSESSMENT

ADMINISTRATIVE

- Set boundaries. What must not be done? What needs to be respected?
- Can you identify any duties or rights that must be respected?
- Autonomy—Maintain respect for persons and the right to self-determination.
- Beneficence—Take note of active suffering that needs to be alleviated. Take note of benefit that can be produced.
- Nonmaleficence—Be wary of creating harm where none exists.
- Justice—Make sure that the interests of the most vulnerable and disadvantaged are acknowledged and respected.
- What maxim describes the relevant policy or plan of action? How does it stand according to the categorical imperative?

STRATEGIC

- Identify the outcomes desired by all people involved in this situation.
- Identify the options available in this situation. (Note: how these options align with the different desired outcomes.)
- For each option, identify the outcomes that can reasonably be anticipated. Conduct a utilitarian analysis.

INTERPERSONAL

- Pay attention to the person you are to care for. What does this person need from you now? How can you help?
- Who has the greatest vulnerability now? Does this person need anything from you? How can you help?
- Who else has needs that you can address? How can you help?
- What about you? What does this situation mean to you? How can you show yourself kindness?

RESULTS

- Gather your own insight from the assessment.
- If possible, discuss your assessment with colleagues and others in position to arrive at a decision on this issue. Strive for consensus wherever possible.

Ethical Assessment Model

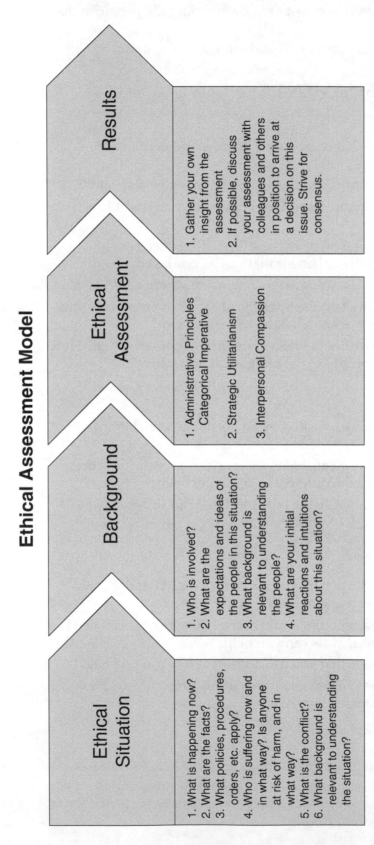

Figure 3.7 Ethical Assessment Model

CASE STUDIES

CASE STUDY 3.1—J-TUBE

Jani is a 4-year-old female, hospitalized with chronic gastritis and other chronic conditions. The gastritis is the reason for her current hospital stay. Her doctors want to bypass her stomach and will place a Jejunostomy tube (J-tube) for nutrition.

Jani's grandmother, Bonnie, is in the hospital room with her. Jani's mother, Marta, has stepped out of the room to get something to eat at the cafeteria. While Marta is out, a resident comes into the room and announces that it's time to place the J-tube. He has a consent form and presents it to Bonnie. The resident goes over the risks and the benefits of the procedure with Bonnie. She signs the form and the resident exits.

An orderly arrives to take Jani to the procedure room. The orderly wheels Jani out of the room, into the hallway and heads toward the elevator when the door opens and Marta steps out. Marta demands to know where Jani is going. A floor nurse steps over and says that Jani is being taken to have her J-tube placed. Marta is angry. She didn't consent to this. The nurse looks at the chart and says, "We have a signed consent form." Marta says, "Well, I didn't sign it!" At this point, Bonnie steps into the hallway, hurries to Marta's side and says, "It's alright, I signed it." Marta is not appeased: "No! It's not your place. I'm her mother! She's my responsibility! It's my right! It's their policy! They have to get consent from me!"

Marta decides to go with Jani to the procedure room so that she can talk to the doctor. Marta intends to make him do another consent form—to do it the right way. Upon arriving at the procedure room, Marta presents her case to the doctor.

Clearly annoyed at Marta's demands and at the fact that she walked into the sterile field, the doctor directs the procedure room nurse to hand Marta a form. Marta accepts the form, signs it, hands it back to the procedure room nurse and walks out. The nurse looks at the form and notices that Marta put the wrong date on the form. She mentions this to the doctor and asks if she should run after Marta. The doctor says, "No. We have a form. Let's go." The nurse further points out that no one explained risks and benefits to Marta. She wasn't properly consented.

Should the procedure continue or should another consent form be signed? Use the Ethical Assessment Model to examine the actions of Marta, Bonnie, the resident, the doctor, the floor nurse, and the procedure room nurse.

CASE STUDY 3.2—DIALYSIS OR COMFORT CARE

Nelson is an 89-year-old male. He has end-stage dementia and is also experiencing kidney failure. Nelson has two daughters, Lauren and Roxanne, each of whom has power of attorney as Nelson's medical surrogate.

Lauren and Roxanne have an appointment with Nelson's doctor. The doctor informs the women that the advancing kidney disease means that they have to make a choice. They can either opt for renal dialysis or they can opt for comfort care. Lauren quickly says that renal dialysis is their choice. She speaks for both of them, confident that Roxanne will be of like mind. Roxanne is not of like mind. She says, "No. Wait. Hasn't Dad been through enough? Maybe it's time . . . ?" Lauren can't believe her ears. Suddenly she doesn't know what to do. Just as suddenly, Roxanne isn't so sure either. They both turn to the doctor and say "What would you do?"

(Continued)

Use the Ethical Assessment Model to evaluate the choice before Lauren and Roxanne. What choice seems best? Use the Ethical Assessment Model to consider how the doctor should respond to Lauren and Roxanne when they ask for advice.

CASE STUDY 3.3—THE DEVOTED DAUGHTER

Prudence is a 32-year-old woman. She is hospitalized with complications due to alcohol withdrawal. Prudence is very ill. She is vomiting and has stomach cramps. She has diarrhea. She is shaking. She is sweating. She is confused. Her nurse, Mack, has a lot on his hands to get her through this.

By Prudence's side is Rossie, her 8-year-old daughter. She is very attentive, even though Prudence is seemingly unaware of her presence. Rossie is sweet, but she is also upset. She has been there all day and hasn't eaten in hours. No one has been able to contact family who can come and get Rossie. She doesn't want to go, anyway. Mack finds that he essentially has two patients. He asks the charge nurse, Lana, if a nursing assistant can watch Rossie and if he can give her a sandwich from the refrigerator. Lana agrees to the first request but says that the only assistant she can spare just went on break and will have to cover the break of another assistant when she returns. In two hours, she can assign an assistant to help with Rossie. As for the sandwich, No. Unit policy states that the food in the refrigerator is for patients only.

Use the Ethical Evaluation Model to explore the options open to Mack. What can he do for Rossie and for Prudence?

REFERENCES

Angel, S., & Vatne, S. (2017). Vulnerability in patients and nurses and the mutual vulnerability in the patient–nurse relationship. *Journal of Clinical Nursing*, 26(9–10), 1428–1437.

Beauchamp, T. L., & Childress, J. F. (2013). *Principles of biomedical ethics* (7th ed., pp. 363–364). New York: Oxford University Press.

Bentham, J. (1996). *An introduction to the principles of morals and legislation*. Oxford: Clarendon Press.

Bloom, P. (2016). *Against empathy: The case for rational compassion*. New York: Ecco.

Broyard, A. (1993). *Intoxicated by my illness: And other writings on life and death*. New York: Fawcett Columbine.

Buchanan, T. W., Bagley, S. L., Stansfield, R. B., & Preston, S. D. (2012). The empathic, physiological resonance of stress. *Social Neuroscience*, 7(2), 191–201.

Charon, R. (2008). *Narrative medicine: Honoring the stories of illness*. New York: Oxford University Press.

Commons, M. L., & Wolfsont, C. A. (2002). A complete theory of empathy must consider stage changes. *Behavioral and Brain Sciences*, 25(1), 30–31.

Conway, K. (2007). *Ordinary life: A memoir of illness*. Ann Arbor: University of Michigan Press.

Decety, J., & Cowell, J. M. (2015). The equivocal relationship between morality and empathy. In J. Decety & T. Wheatley (Eds.). *The moral brain: A multidisciplinary perspective* (pp. 279–302). Cambridge, MA: MIT Press.

EPA. (n.d.). *Selected EPA-registered disinfectants*. Northwest, Washington, D.C.: Environmental Protection Agency. Retrieved from https://www.epa.gov/pesticide-registration/selected-epa-registered-disinfectants

Fies, B. (2008). *Mom's cancer.* New York: Abrams Comicarts.

Frank, A. W. (2013). *The wounded storyteller: Body, illness, and ethics.*

Frankfurt, H. G. (2010). *On bullshit.* Princeton, NJ: Princeton University Press.

Gilbert, P. (2017). Compassion: definitions and controversies. In P. Gilbert (Ed.). *Compassion: concepts, research and applications.* London/New York/Routledge: Taylor & Francis.

Gruen, L. (2009). Attending to nature: Empathetic engagement with the more than human world. *Ethics & the Environment, 14*(2): 23–38.

Hall, B. A. (2005). *The art of becoming a nurse healer.* Orlando, FL: Bandido Books.

Host, C. (2011). *Between me and the river: Living beyond cancer: A memoir.* New York: Harlequin.

Kant, I. (1960). *Religion within the limits of reason alone* (T. M. Greene & H. H. Hudson, Trans.). New York: Harper and Brothers.

Kant, I. (2010). *Grounding for the metaphysics of morals: With on a supposed right to lie because of philanthropic concerns.* Indianapolis, IN: Hackett Publishing Company.

Keen, S. (2006). A theory of narrative empathy. *Narrative, 14*(3), 207–236.

Loggia, M. L., Mogil, J. S., & Catherine, B. M. (2008). Empathy hurts: Compassion for another increases both sensory and affective components of pain perception. *Pain, 136,* 168–176.

Lorde, A. (2006). *The cancer journals.* San Francisco, CA: Aunt Lutes Books.

Martin, L. J., Hathaway, G., Isbester, K., Mirali, S., Acland, E. L., Niederstrasser, N. . . . Mogil, J. S. (2015). Reducing social stress elicits emotional contagion of pain in mouse and human strangers. *Current Biology, 25*(3), 326–332.

Middlebrook, C. (1998). *Seeing the crab: A memoir of dying before I do.* New York: Anchor Books.

Mill, J. S (1998). *Utilitarianism.* Oxford: Oxford University Press.

NIOSH-CDC. (2018). Bloodborne infectious diseases: HIV/AIDS, Hepatitis B, Hepatitis C. Atlanta, GA: Centers for Disease Control and Prevention. Retrieved from https://www.cdc.gov/niosh/topics/bbp/

NMTCB. (2012). *Code of ethics.* Tucker, GA: Nuclear Medicine Technology Certification Board. Retrieved from https://www.nmtcb.org/policies/ethics.php

OSHA. (n.d.). *Bloodborne pathogens: Occupational safety and health standards.* Washington, DC: Occupational Safety and Health Administration. Retrieved from https://www.osha.gov/pls/oshaweb/owadisp.show_document?p_table=standards&p_id=10051.

Prinz, J. (2011). Is empathy necessary for morality. In A. Coplan & P. Goldie (Eds.). *Empathy: philosophical and psychological perspectives.* New York: Oxford University Press 211–229.

Radner, G. (2009). *It's always something.* New York: Simon & Schuster Paperbacks.

Śāntideva. (2008). *The way of the Bodhisattva* (p. 48). Boston, MA: Shambhala Publication.

Sinclair, S., McClement, S., Raffin-Bouchal, S., Hack, T. F., Hagen, N. A., McConnell, S., Chochinov, H. M. (2016). Compassion in health care: An empirical model. *Journal of Pain and Symptom Management, 51*(2), 193–203.

Skloot, R. (2010). *The immortal life of Henrietta Lacks.* New York: Crown Publishers.

Thich Nhat Hanh. (1998). *The vows of the four great Bodhisattvas.* Dharma Talk given by Thich Nhat Hanh on January 15, 1998 in Plum Village, France. Retrieved from http://www.buddhist-canon.com/PUBLIC/PUBNOR/NHATHANH/1998%20Jan%2015%20%20The%20Four%20Great%20Bodhisattva%20Vows.htm

van der Cingel, M. (2011). Compassion in care: A qualitative study of older people with a chronic disease and nurses. *Nursing Ethics, 18*(5), 672–685.

Watson, J. (2008). *Nursing: The philosophy and science of caring.* Boulder, CO: University Press of Colorado.

PROFESSIONAL INTEGRITY

OBJECTIVES

After completing this chapter, you will be able to . . .

1. Describe the nature of integrity and its relationship with virtue.

2. Describe Aristotle's ethics on all three levels of ethical assessment. Apply Aristotle's theory to efforts to develop character.

3. Identify the concept of professional integrity and discuss how it applies in practice.

4. Examine and compare professional oaths.

5. Apply the levels of ethical assessment to codes of ethics.

6. Describe ethical relativism and examine its impact on a professional oath and code of ethics.

7. Identify the function and characteristics of a role model.

8. Apply the Ethical Assessment Model to chapter exercises and to real-life scenarios.

KEY TERMS

- Character
- Code of ethics
- Ethical relativism
- Eudaimonia
- Fiduciary

- Integrity
- Oath
- Role model
- Tolerance
- Virtue

Physical therapists shall demonstrate integrity in their relationships with patients/clients, families, colleagues, students, research participants, other health care providers, employers, payers, and the public (Core Value: Integrity) (APTA, 2013).

INTRODUCTION

Integrity is a condition of virtue in which the self is whole, harmonious, and intact.

A professional who has integrity can be counted on to uphold the standards of the profession. This is more than just following orders and doing your job. **Integrity** is wholeness. There is predictability and trustworthiness. Integrity includes the predictability that someone will adhere to policy and regulation, respecting rights and dignity. It includes the trust that someone will follow proper procedure and protocol, working for the best outcomes as per the function of the profession. The professional who has integrity will be reliable and consistent in upholding the tasks and standards of the profession. Conscientious choice will be made to uphold these standards and perform the tasks of the role.

Conscientious choice involves devotion to your role, to your tasks, and to how you express yourself in this role and through these tasks. In this way, integrity is a matter of character—of knowing that someone has embraced the function of the professional role as a matter of character and as an expression of that person.

Character refers to those qualities and attributes in a human being that marks one's reliability for moral behavior.

The word **character** is derived from a Greek word that is used to name a stamping tool, which could be used, for instance, to stamp a value on a coin. In this sense, character referred to something that stood out about a coin, identifying it and marking its value. When we incorporate character into ethics, we have in mind that which stands out about an individual as a demonstration of the person's moral qualities and attributes. Your character is the value you show through your actions.

Character refers to something that is central to who you are and how you move through your life. It points to that which is consistently expressed in how you think, how you act, and who you find yourself to be. What you consistently do shows your character. Your character points back to you. Other people can anticipate certain actions and behaviors from you based upon what they have observed from you before. This is what others will understand and describe as your character.

It is important to acknowledge that character can change. None of us are the same as we were 5 years ago. Character changes with experience, circumstances, social interactions, life events, aging, and other factors. You don't just sit back and watch your character change over time. You are involved in this process. Ethically, you hold the expectation that you *should* be involved in this process; that you have responsibility for your character.

Professional integrity revolves around taking responsibility for your character. Understand your role and understand that this role belongs to you. See the value in your role and in doing it well. Your activity in this role is a way of expressing your character.

Professional integrity means taking this responsibility to mold your character into one that embraces the core activity of the profession. You identify with your profession. In your profession, there is a standard to uphold. Professional standards minimize risks, reflecting an interest in avoiding harm. They establish predictability. There are people you can count on to be compassionate. They are reliable. This is character.

Reputation is a reflection of character. It is the way your signature style is portrayed. It is how other people would describe you. It is not what you look like; it is what you act like. Reputation is more than what other people think of you. It is also what you think of yourself.

EXERCISE

Describe a person in your life whom you admire. How do you describe this person? Is your description informed by how this person looks or by how this person acts? Next, think about the way you describe other people—strangers, patients, and coworkers. Do you describe them according to the way they look or according to the way they act?

Your reputation, then, presents you with choices. How do you see yourself? Who should you be? How will you act in order to see yourself as the person you want to be? Choices like these can bring you to think about what it means to be your best self. What does it mean to be whole? To have integrity?

INTEGRITY

Take a moment to think about integrity. What comes to mind? Honesty is frequently associated with integrity. But do we really mean this? Do we want to say that someone has integrity if they speak what they believe is true even if they callously disregard the feelings of others as they speak their minds? Do we say that someone has integrity if they honestly profess their opinions, even though they are badly misinformed?

Honesty is one way to approach integrity, but there must be more. Indeed, the etymology of the word integrity suggests that it carries the meaning of being intact, of being whole. Honesty is one trait that might contribute to the person you feel you ought to be. This ideal version of yourself will have other admirable traits as well. By itself, honesty might not be enough to reliably guide you to good action, but in harmony with other traits—within the overall wholeness of a person possessing integrity—honesty can stand out as one quality among several of an exceptional human being.

Wholeness has an organic quality. To show this, first contrast a whole with a totality. A totality is a mere aggregation of parts. Lump various things together. Aggregated together, these things now constitute a totality; there is no reason for them to be together, but they now fit with each other loosely. You may have some purpose in bringing them together, but there is no natural—internal—reason for them to belong with each other. The human body, on the other hand, is a whole. It is a collection of various parts that all fit together, work together, and influence each other. You've learned this in the study of anatomy and physiology. These organs and tissues constitute a whole. They work together according to some internal process, which is the life and growth of the body.

Each organ has its function that it contributes to the whole. The whole—the organism—then has a fundamental activity that is made possible by the work of all these organs. Homeostasis among the various parts of the body facilitates health and growth. In all organisms, there is at least this purpose—to grow vigorously.

We do not adequately understand the whole human being simply by acknowledging the organs of the body and the manner in which they interact and promote homeostasis. We have body and mind. Just as organs, tissues, and cells have roles in homeostasis in the body, so qualities of the person contribute to the wholeness—the integrity—of the self. Wholeness is not just staying together as you are. It is especially a matter of growth—of performing well and of continuing to develop in competence and influence.

Homeostasis is integrity of the organism. But the being—the human being—is more than that. Growth for us includes our social and intellectual lives, as well as our physical health. Integrity for us, then, involves the application of our mind and our passions toward the fundamental activity of being human. **Virtue** is excellence at these activities.

Virtue is excellence of character, or excellence in character traits.

This integrity is excellence in the fundamental activity of a human being. A good person will be one who acts with virtue. When it comes to professions, there is a fundamental activity that distinguishes the professional from those outside the profession. Excellence in this activity is professional integrity.

ARISTOTLE AND INTEGRITY

The three levels of ethical assessment are meant to offer a way to approach the complexity of our moral and social lives. They are tools to help us to discern and clarify what is at stake as we face morally challenging issues.

Normative ethical theories are designed with this sort of usefulness in mind. Even though we associated several normative theories in Chapter 3 with one level of ethical assessment, each will have its way of applying toward other levels of assessment. Students and scholars of moral philosophy will have looked at Chapter 3 and noted one glaring omission. *Aristotle! Where is Aristotle?* We reserve Aristotle for this chapter. More than reserving his ethical theory for a spotlight here, we offer Aristotle as an example of a theorist who strongly captures the three levels of ethical assessment. As he did so, Aristotle also presented a compelling way of capturing professional integrity.

To be precise, Aristotle never mentioned professionalism. His focus was on humanity. Aristotle identified the highest good—that which is worth seeking for its own sake and not for the sake of bringing about something else—as *eudaimonia*. Translations of Aristotle often render eudaimonia as *happiness*. This can work, but it will be misleading if we associate happiness with pleasure. You might think of someone who experiences pleasure and hurts others in the process. Such a person, you might believe, does not deserve to be happy. Eudaimonia would not include such pleasure. This is a moral concept that emphasizes the overall character of the person (Aristotle, 2002).

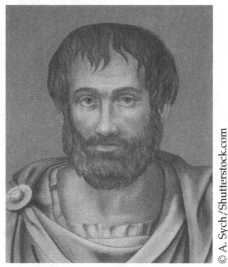

Figure 4.1 Aristotle

A more literal translation of **eudaimonia** is *having a good spirit*. To experience eudaimonia—to be virtuously happy—is to possess integrity. Ethically speaking, eudaimonia is the state of living the good life, of knowing that you are experiencing a life well lived. As an experience, integrity is not merely what you do. Integrity belongs to the character of one who reliably acts as a person ought to act. A good action here and there does not make for eudaimonia. It takes a character—a spirit—from which good actions are chosen on an everyday basis.

Eudaimonia is the Aristotelian concept of the highest state of virtue.

EXERCISE

Eudaimonia is commonly translated as happiness. A better way to think of it is as having a good spirit, having integrity. Think about this. What do you see as the relationship between happiness and integrity?

On an administrative-level view, virtue in general is excellence in the functioning of attributes that are characteristic of a human being. The virtuous person exhibits behavior that reflects excellence of character. In Aristotle's view, humans are characterized by their capacity for rational thought. So, virtue entails reasoning well. If we could measure integrity as the administrative level in the Aristotelian sense, we would assess how closely a person approximates an ideal of a rational person. But it is not enough to reason abstractly; we must reason well in our daily activity (Aristotle, 2002).

Recognizing that we are passionate beings as well as rational, Aristotle held that virtuous action entails a rational effort to bring harmony to the emotional states that can motivate our actions. Our passions, when experienced in excess, can motivate us to react to aspects of our circumstances before we properly assess what we face. Our passions, when experienced in deficiency, also can demotivate us from engaging circumstances that are deserving of our attention.

This, then, is the strategic level of Aristotelian ethics: mustering a rational effort to moderate our passions between the extremes of excess and deficiency and toward a mean state. Courage, for instance, is a virtuous attitude toward taking personal risks. It is a moderate position between foolhardiness (excessive risk taking) and cowardice (deficient risk taking). Were we to measure integrity at this level in the Aristotelian sense, we would assess specific actions and test them against the strategic method of rationally guiding passions into the mean state between extremes (Aristotle, 2002).

To take another example, Aristotle described generosity as a virtue involving two concerns: giving and receiving wealth. Wastefulness is excessive in giving and spending. It can also involve deficiency in earning or receiving wealth. Greed or stinginess is the opposite. It is deficient in spending while excessive in desiring to accumulate wealth (Aristotle, 2002).

Aristotle's strategic model asks you to reflect on yourself before you reflect on your situation. *What is motivating me in this situation? What would excessive passion be like for me right now? What would deficient passion be like for me? How can I moderate my passion between these?* This strategic process steers us toward virtue in several ways. First, the process engages your rational mind in your daily activity. You act all day on motivations that naturally arise within you, influenced by your passions. This process asserts a harmonizing place for your rational mind in the way these emotions arise. Second, as your rational mind steers your passions toward a moderate condition, you act more virtuously. Third, the more you are able to act virtuously with consistency, the more you develop habits of virtue. The more your virtues become your habits, the more virtue takes root deep within you as a matter of character.

Finally, integrity is revealed and fed in relationships between persons. The topic that receives the most attention in Aristotle's

Nicomachean Ethics is friendship. In friendship, Aristotle addresses the interpersonal level of ethics. Here, we find a bond between two people who, in the best expression of friendship, wish that the other person experiences what is good. This is to say that friends of the best sort take an interest in the integrity of each other. Friends will engage each other rationally, both intellectually and in moral fellowship. You can call attention to your friend's habits and behaviors, just as you should be open to honest and forthright assessment from your friend (Aristotle, 2002).

Aristotle notes that friendship creates stronger bonds than abstract ideals of justice. Justice serves well to drive policies, laws, and considerations of rights. But in friendship, your own sense of self expands to include the other. You have concern for your friend as you have concern for yourself. This bond is more than abstract. Virtue is not simply an ideal here; it is practiced and lived. Justice, like eudaimonia, calls you like a distant, guiding star. Friendship, however, needs your present and active attention.

ARISTOTELIAN ETHICS AND THE LEVELS OF ASSESSMENT		
ADMINISTRATIVE LEVEL	STRATEGIC LEVEL	INTERPERSONAL LEVEL
Eudaimonia	Virtuous behavior as rationally steering passions between the extremes of excess or deficiency	Friendship

Figure 4.2 Aristotelian Ethics and the Levels of Ethical Assessment

Through Aristotle's ethics, we traced the three levels of ethical assessment. In Chapter 3, we examined each level separately. Here, we can see how one may theoretically engage all three levels. Further, Aristotle's ethics enables us to view integrity from the perspective of each of these three levels. Administratively, integrity is wholeness of the person, a fulfillment and perfection of character. Strategically, integrity is a project, crafted through a procedural approach to decision-making. Interpersonally, integrity is manifest in the relationship with another, in which both parties are invested in the welfare and growth of each other.

Aristotle addressed integrity for humanity as a whole and for human beings in their daily lives. From here, we will examine integrity as it is specific to a profession. Just as your integrity as a person involves wholeness in the fundamental activity of being human, so professional integrity involves wholeness in the activities essential to your profession. Implicit in this approach to integrity is the association of virtue with the essential performance of your work as a professional. In other words, ethical competency is promoted as a necessary part of your work.

THE GOOD OF VIRTUE

It's understandable if, in your training, your attention diverts to learning other knowledge bases and skill sets. As a student, developing clinical competency is critical to passing your classes and gaining licensure. Clinical competency will require you to take in new information and learn new skills. Virtue isn't required in order to obtain your professional license. You'll need to show some awareness of ethics as you obtain your license, but you won't have to demonstrate that you are virtuous in order to become licensed. And you already have your moral beliefs. You can sort out right from wrong. You might honestly feel that you have bigger things to worry about.

Yet, as seen in the first two chapters of this text, morality is easy until it isn't. Your moral beliefs make sense to you, but only because they arise according to the limits of your own perspective. Other perspectives are possible; when you are in position to consider the views of others it becomes necessary to go outside the comfort of your own view. Being a professional means taking on the interests of others—patients—who need your services. These patients will have their own perspectives. Your work as a professional will also mean that you will collaborate with other professionals and interact with members of the public—all of whom will have somewhat different perspectives from you. As a professional, you will operate within a regulated industry with policies and procedures that set boundaries and provide guidance for your behavior. These policies and procedures are set according to perspectives that might differ from your own. Put simply, your work as a professional will involve moral complications that will place your ethical competency to the test. Virtue, therefore, aligns with all aspects of your work as a professional.

What you do as a professional has to benefit others. The reason for the profession is to provide needed services that others cannot provide for themselves. This service brings you into contact with others in their vulnerability, and so your service carries a risk of harm. There are many things in place to protect patients. Policies, regulations, procedures, and protocols. There are disincentives to act in such a way as to harm patients—fines and license suspensions, for instance. In some way, the patient's best protection is your virtue. A virtuous character will make patient safety a conscientious choice. The virtuous professional is motivated by desire to protect and benefit the patient.

Imagine that you are a professional and you enter a patient's room during a periodic hand-hygiene audit. Someone watches health-care members enter and exit rooms in this unit. This person will report on anyone who touches a patient without proper hand washing. You wash your hands as you enter the room. Why? Are you primarily motivated to wash your hands because you don't want to get in trouble or because you have been ordered to? Or, do you wash your hands because doing so is good for your patient? Which is the better motivation? Virtue means embracing the tasks and purposes of your role, recognizing the worth in doing them. The virtuous professional will be motivated more by the worth of the role and its tasks than by any external incentives to behave well.

Virtue is good for all and maintains the integrity of the profession. Virtue promotes better outcomes. Virtue positions you to be of benefit to those with whom you are in direct contact. And reciprocally, all of these goods can come back to benefit you. Virtue brings you benefit as your virtuous behavior contributes to the growth of your character.

Ethics is what you do. Virtue is who you are. The two really can't be distinguished. Who you are informs what you'll do. And what you do reveals who you are. This means taking an interest in integrity. Since your integrity at work will entail wholeness in the essential tasks of your profession, it is important to turn our attention now to the nature of a profession and to professional virtues. The goal is to develop the skills to know the kind of conduct you need to cultivate and to find a way to exhibit that conduct.

ETHICS AND THE ART OF BEING A PROFESSIONAL

A profession is a vocation that offers a valued service. The professional has a background in education and practice that contribute to the possession of expertise that is both uncommon and needed. The professional possesses a knowledge and skill-base that is not held by most people.

The professional enters into a **fiduciary** relationship with clients. Such a relationship is based upon vulnerability and trust. The client is made vulnerable by some pressing need. In health care, of course, we have in mind patients. Patients are made vulnerable by illness, injury, or by the threat of illness or injury, and the devastations that illness or injury can wreak on one's life. Patients do not have the capacity to treat their own illness or injury, and so they are made more vulnerable. Needing help, patients turn to health-care professionals for aid. It is these professionals who possess the necessary skills and expertise to effectively come to the patient's aid. This is to say that the patient remains vulnerable unless and until health-care professionals provide needed treatment. Patients are in a position in which they are compelled to trust the professionals whom they seek out for treatment. Professional integrity brings a heightened expectation of a virtue to be trustworthy. Supporting trustworthy behaviors is a central part of professional integrity in health care.

Patients who seek out health-care professionals have an expectation of care. In this interaction between patient and professional, care will be guided by policy and procedure. Policies are in place to protect. Procedures are in place to direct treatment toward patient outcomes. In

Fiduciary describes a relationship, such as a professional relationship, that is built on trust.

addition to guidelines like these, there are also expectations that extend from professional virtue. Policy, procedure, and virtue all belong within the expectations of professional standards.

A professional belongs to an organization that establishes standards of competence that set expectations for knowledge, technical performance, and conduct. Standards of competence include some attention to fiduciary duties that professionals have toward their clients. Those clients will also have their own conception of the profession and expectations of the professional. In some measure, the expectations of the client are influenced by cultural assumptions about professions in general and about the professional's particular field.

In other words, a professional is expected to hold a set of competencies. Standards for those competencies are variously set by the professional organization, by individual clients and by the broader culture(s) of the client and professional. These expectations might not always align with each other. People outside of a profession—such as patients and other members of the public—view members of a profession in a way that might not align with the way professionals understand what it means to live and practice their craft.

The popular conception of professionals is built around the common assumption that a professional possesses a heightened moral character and quality of spirit. Professionals have a responsibility to treat patients within the scope of their professional abilities. Patients, then, should be able to trust their health-care professionals within the boundaries of the provision of care. However, patients might assume that the trust they extend to the professional for care of illness or injury also extends to trust in the professional's overall character as a human being. Patients might also assume that professionals have a valued social status with a level of compensation and lifestyle to match. Many professionals are fortunate enough to have such elevated acclaim and prosperity, but this is not universally true of all professionals (Becker, 1962).

Clients might hold assumptions that the professionals they work with meet cultural expectations. The expectations of clients can also be shaped by the reason why a fiduciary relationship with a professional is sought in the first place—need. The client has particular need of the expertise held by the professional. Inherently, then, there is an imbalance in the power structure between client and professional. The client needs more service from the professional than the professional needs from the client. If the professional neglects to serve the client, the client can be harmed—in many cases irreparably. The professional will typically have many clients while the client will often have few, or just this one, professionals to serve this particular need. Hence, the client may feel vulnerable with respect to the professional and somewhat in awe of the professional's perceived status, ability, and advantage over the client. In this position, clients may approach the professional with mislaid trust. They might expect miracles. These expectations could turn to feelings of betrayal if miracles do not ensue. In contrast, clients might feel intimidation at the status of the professional and approach the professional with a mixture of fear, suspicion, jealousy, and contempt. In short, the expectations of the client may be out of pace with the professional's own self-image based on personal and professional perspectives.

Despite differences in their expectations, patients still have worth. Recognize the personal value of each person. Each patient has the same value abstractly but must be valued individually for the unique persons that they are. Find the value in what you do and in who you are as a professional.

Patients vary. Circumstances vary. Orders vary. Day to day shifts will change. What doesn't vary are the standards for professional virtue. These standards will be reflected in one's professional oath and code of ethics.

PROFESSIONAL OATHS

An **oath** is a promise. It is a personal testament. It is a self-declaration that you will hold yourself to a standard of behavior and character. An oath is therefore an act of authenticity in which you determine who you will be. You alone are responsible for taking the oath and for living up to the promise. Your oath is your own. Once made it can't be taken away except by your own choice and action. Failing your oath means abandoning a vision you once declared of who you will be.

All oaths are personal. Some of them are also professional. You self-identify who you need to be as a member of the profession you will soon enter. An oath is also a reminder. Before stepping into the professional arena, it is a way of aligning yourself with the demands, expectations, and ideals that come with your role.

> An **oath** is a vow or promise that makes a declaration about one's future behavior and can serve as a guide.

EXERCISE

There are other oaths that people take. Many marriage ceremonies including the taking of oaths (wedding vows). Aside from professional oaths, what other oaths do people take? What is the function or purpose of taking an oath? What makes an oath meaningful?

One of the best-known professional oaths is the *Hippocratic Oath*. This is exclusive to doctors. Here we can see the pledge taken by doctors and compare it to a common oath taken by nurses at their pinning ceremony. We can get some sense of the perspectives taken by doctors and nurses. What do the differences in the oaths suggest about the potential for differences in perspective taken by members of the professions?

The Hippocratic Oath is one of the oldest known oaths. As such, speaking it perhaps gives many medical school graduates a feeling of continuity with an ancient and honored tradition. However, because it is ancient, the Hippocratic Oath contains language and provisions that no longer capture the demands and concerns of the modern-day physician. For that reason, many medical schools use modernized versions of the oath. Here is one such version, written in 1964 by Louis Lasagna of the School of Medicine at Tufts University (Lasagna, 1964).

For comparison, here is the Florence Nightingale Pledge. This was created in 1893 by a committee at the Farrand School for Nursing. The committee, led by Lystra Gretter, modeled the pledge after the Hippocratic Oath. It was revised in 1935.

I solemnly pledge myself before God and in the presence of this assembly, to pass my life in purity and to practice my profession faithfully. I will abstain from whatever is deleterious and mischievous and will not take or knowingly administer any harmful drug. I will do all in my power to maintain and elevate the standard of my profession and will hold in confidence all personal matters committed to my keeping, and all family affairs coming to my knowledge in the practice of my calling. With loyalty will I endeavor to aid the physician in his work, and as a 'missioner of health' I will dedicate myself to devoted service to human welfare.

Source: McBurney and Filoromo (1994).

EXERCISE

Compare the Florence Nightingale Pledge with the Hippocratic Oath. How does each oath fit its respective profession? What important similarities and differences do you see?

There are other versions of this nursing pledge. An oath can be modified for its time, its culture, or its audience. An oath is not simply a vehicle to carry a statement of virtues and mission. It should have meaning for those who profess this oath. The phrasing of an oath can be adjusted so that it can speak to those who are taking it. Here is a pledge from the International Council of Nurses:

> *In the full knowledge of the task I am undertaking, I promise to take care of the sick with all the skill and understanding I possess, without regard to race, creed, color, politics, or social status, sparing no effort to conserve life, to alleviate suffering, and promote health.*
>
> *I will respect at all times the dignity and religious beliefs of the patients entrusted in my care, holding in confidence all personal information entrusted to me and refraining from any action which might endanger life or health.*
>
> *I will endeavor to keep my professional knowledge and skill at the highest level and give loyal support and cooperation to all members of the health team.*
>
> *I will do my utmost to honor the international code of ethics applied to nursing and to uphold the integrity of the nurse.*
>
> *Source*: de Tornyay (1989).

As you utter your oath, you declare your fundamental professional intentions to those who stand in witness. At the same time, your oath is speaking to you.

Exercise

Compare these versions of the Nurse's Pledge. What are the core ideas that remain the same in these pledges? Do you also find these core ideas in the Hippocratic Oath? Write your own version of the Nightingale Pledge that captures these core ideas and also is especially meaningful to you.

Your oath is for you. An oath strives to capture a spirit and a motivation in choosing to join a profession. When you start feeling cynical or abandoned, go back to your oath. Read your oath. It's a way to bring you back toward center. Your oath can be a reminder of what it's all about. Back to your autonomy. You chose this professional pathway. Think of why. Think of all that is involved with this pathway.

EXERCISE

Read the Florence Nightingale Pledge and the Hippocratic Oath from the perspective of Aristotelian ethics. What virtues are promoted in each oath? How will Aristotelian ethics help a new nurse or doctor cultivate the virtues identified in these oaths?

The professional code of ethics is for everyone. The code of ethics overlaps with policy, regulation, education, and job standards. Codes of ethics point to areas in which professional conduct can be evaluated and judged.

CODES OF ETHICS

A **code of ethics** is a document that outlines the core mission, principles, and virtues of an organization or profession.

Codes of ethics try to preserve what it takes to stay whole. This is why they have the scope that they do. Think about your code of ethics. Just as you should see the value in your patient, see the value in your oath and in your code of ethics. How can this guide you to integrity?

The provisions in a code of ethics can come across as obvious and, therefore, not interesting. This is the appearance that comes from the direct expression of the standards. But ethics comes into play when circumstances become complicated and confusing—when we don't know what to do or when we find conflict.

An event of ethical significance is when we have to think about what is happening and what we ought to do. The path from a clearly expressed standard to action and interpersonal connection is harder to discern. The clear standards of a code of ethics can be a light to guide in the fog. It might be easy to take the standards of a code of ethics for granted, as we assume that we are good people who just know how to behave. It's in situations where we face uncertainty, that reflecting on the values in the code are especially necessary. The code of ethics supports, validates, and facilitates critical thinking and ethical decision-making.

EXERCISE

Find a Code of Ethics from another allied health profession and from a profession not directly related to health care. Compare the provisions of each code. What similarities and differences do you note? What does your comparison reveal to you about the differences between these professions?

There is real meaning to a code of ethics. Pointing to professional integrity, the code of ethics orients toward wholeness. All three levels of ethical assessment can be engaged. To demonstrate, four codes of ethics for nurses are presented here. Each will be examined in a different way for the purpose of illustrating a different objective.

FOUR CODES OF ETHICS AS EXAMPLES

Four codes of ethics for the nursing profession will be explored here. These are from the American Nurses Association, the International Council of Nurses, The Japanese Nurses Association, and the Canadian Nurses Association. We will use these codes from the same profession to facilitate your comparison. Each professional organization offers its own interpretive comments. What follows here will be an exercise in reading each code from the perspective of our three levels of ethical assessment.

AMERICAN NURSES ASSOCIATION (ANA) CODE OF ETHICS

First, consider the code of ethics from the American Association of Nurses (ANA) which will be presented and read to derive direction for all three levels of assessment. There are nine provisions to the ANA Code of Ethics. These provisions address nursing competencies with respect to standards that are to be upheld between the nurse and various stakeholders in the profession. The most obvious and vulnerable stakeholder is the patient. Fittingly the first three provisions specify ethical standards of care toward patients. Provision 4 addresses standards for the nurse's conduct and competencies at work. Provision 5 addresses the nurse's obligations to self—to be the best person and best nurse possible. Provisions 6 and 7 address the nurse's role in contributing to the development of the profession and to medical science. Provisions 8 and 9 address the nurse's role in society as an advocate for health for all.

1. **The nurse practices with compassion and respect for the inherent dignity, worth, and unique attributes of every person.**

   Interpersonal—The ANA Code of ethics doesn't open with skills or level of education. It is all-encompassing. And compassion is listed first! This is the prime virtue. Nursing emphasizes the interpersonal.

   Strategic—Attention to detail is important. The plan of care is specific to the patient. This is the one thing that you can individualize to the patient. It identifies the individuality of the patient's needs and treatments. It's how you target a good outcome.

   Administrative—Respect for dignity. In the Kantian sense, dignity entails respecting each person as a rational being. Even if your patients aren't being rational, you still treat them with dignity. They're sick and they're scared, but you still treat them as dignified beings.

2. **The nurse's primary commitment is to the patient, whether an individual, family, group, community, or population.**

   Interpersonal—When patients are in distress, they call out for the nurse. They know that it is the nurse who will meet that cry. Patients and families reach out to the one who they know is going to respond. The person you work with directly receives your care.

   Strategic—This is the level of clinical care. Here is the dedication to use your clinical skills and to demonstrate commitment to bring about health outcomes. This also includes your dedication to develop your expertise and maintain your knowledge for your skill set. At this level you can see where your work directly contributes to health outcomes.

   Administrative—This level conceives of health for a community or population. When policies are set, bear in mind who they are to benefit. When policies are drafted, they are not intended for a particular patient or professional. They are global in scope. In adhering to a policy, recognize the value in contributing to an all-encompassing effort to promote health.

3. **The nurse promotes, advocates for, and protects the rights, health, and safety of the patient.**

   Interpersonal—This is the way a nurse compassionately delivers care. It makes a difference when patients know that their nurse listens to them and advocates for them.

   Strategic—Following procedures, protocols and orders, the nurse provides predictability of care. The nurse is present to offer interventions to relieve the patient's suffering.

   Administrative—Many policies are in place for the purpose of protecting patients' rights and to protect patients from harm.

4. **The nurse has authority, accountability, and responsibility for nursing practice; makes decisions; and takes action consistent with the obligation to promote health and to provide optimal care.**

   Interpersonal—Compassionate action needs to be responsive to the patient's needs. The willingness to pay attention to the patient brings responsibility to serve the needs of the patient as a person, as one who suffers.

   Strategic—Nursing practice is a collaborative effort. Each person in this effort has roles and duties that contribute to health outcomes.

   Administrative—You're not alone in taking responsibility for the care you give to your patients. There is an expectation that you follow policies for the safety of patients and the public. Following policy also protects the nurse.

5. **The nurse has a duty to self to maintain competence and to continue professional growth.**

   Interpersonal—This provision points to the importance of cultivating wholeness. It's your responsibility to maintain and promote your professional integrity. Integrity doesn't only mean practicing self-restraint. An important part of integrity is self-compassion. This is the direction of thought in identifying your own needs as a professional and as a person. It is a matter of regrouping. Self-compassion isn't limited to relaxation techniques. It's fine to treat yourself to a massage, but you have needs beyond relaxation. Positioning yourself to be skilled and competent in your profession helps you to grow and to have the satisfaction from helping those in need and from being good at your job.

   Strategic—These are the opportunities you chose to continue professional growth, continuing education. You make these choices for the purpose of staying current with skills and practice.

   Administrative—Professional organizations and employers will provide opportunities for professional development, but it's up to your integrity to avail yourself of the opportunities. In Chapter 3, we saw that Immanuel Kant spoke of the moral permissibility of self-improvement. It is for each of us to find the right time, place, and opportunity to pursue self-improvement. Professionally, the opportunities are there. Your duty extends to taking advantage of such opportunities to grow and enhance your ability to fulfill your professional role.

6. **The nurse facilitates improvement of the health-care environment.**

   Interpersonal—Environments are complex. We interact and engage people in many different ways. We offer the three levels of ethical assessment because we find these different levels of interaction and perception in our lives. On the interpersonal level, we impact our health-care environment through one-on-one contact. Whether working with a patient, a family member, or a coworker, you get a response from compassionate interaction. This interaction can make all the difference, improving the health-care environment in that small but significant space.

Strategic—At this level, there is concern for patient outcomes and safety. Your observations can contribute to evidence-based development of the protocols that shape the moral environment. Communication and collaboration are essential to a process in which protocols can be improved and disseminated. With effective communication, a flow of patient care can be maintained. Communication and collaboration are also essential to a culture in which professionals can work with respect and support.

Administrative—It is easy to become overwhelmed when we contemplate improving an environment as a whole. The most direct way to improve an overall health-care environment is by crafting policies and regulations. You can facilitate improvement in the moral environment where you work by following the policies that are in place. More, you have the responsibility to be aware of how well these policies serve this moral environment. Use the Ethical Assessment Model as a way to explore the value in policies that are set for you. If the model leads you to see that there is room for improvement, then you might be able to see out opportunities to serve on committees that review and establish policies.

7. **The nurse assists in advancement of the profession through contributions to practice, education, administration, and knowledge development.**

   Interpersonal—Situational awareness has educational value. Pay attention to what people need. In your interactions with patients, families, and coworkers with your own self-awareness—what is needed? Where can we do better? And how can we use practice, education, and so on. to help find ways to make things better at the bedside?

   Strategic—At this level you contribute to learning in the clinical and classroom settings. You will have opportunities to make your contributions both as a student and as an instructor. There is value in being a student because there is purpose in the knowledge and skills you pursue. There are known duties to pursue education: completing the coursework necessary to graduate and completing continuing education credits. As you pursue your education, there is self-declaration of your devotion to be a nurse. There are opportunities to be an instructor. These opportunities include patient education, public education, and mentoring student nurses.

Administrative—Nursing practice is not stagnant; it is dynamic. Nursing education must be dynamic as well. You can contribute to the development of nursing education. You can support education in many ways: You can subscribe to professional journals or participate in conferences or in research. You can participate in regional or state committees and boards.

8. **The nurse collaborates with the public and other health professionals in promoting community, national, and international efforts to meet health needs.**

    Interpersonal—Each patient you encounter is vulnerable in some way. Attending to your patient as a trustworthy and compassionate professional elevates the dignity of that patient.

    Strategic—A right to health can be endorsed by aligning with the practice of nursing. Nursing is a profession devoted to meeting health needs. Doing your job affirms each patient as deserving of your care. You might also have opportunities to act professionally to address specific issues of social justice. For instance, you might have the chance to take your practice to underserved communities that are in particular need.

    Administrative—There is no right to be healthy. Injury or illness can happen to us all. When we speak of a right to health, we speak of access to health care and to other goods that are necessary to the promotion of health. Nurses can lead and participate in community education health awareness programs. Nurses can also lead and participate in efforts to bring needed care to underserved regions.

9. **The profession of nursing collectively through its professional organizations, must articulate nursing values, maintain the integrity of the profession, and integrate principles of social justice into nursing and health policy.**

    Interpersonal—You don't engage interpersonally with a society. You engage interpersonally with another individual. Justice, at this level, is an abstract consideration. The reality is the person in front of you. Understand your professional role and expectations. Pay attention to the person before you. Your compassionate action will affirm the dignity of that person. In this small space, there is justice—there is something stronger, more tangible even than justice.

    Strategic—Here you become involved, taking a stand for justice for those who suffer disparities in health and access to health care. There are many ways to do this. You can volunteer your time, raise awareness, engage in activism. The purpose of your involvement is goal-driven, much like the clinical effort to bring about health outcomes for a patient. Now, though, your purpose is to contribute to an effort to bring about desired social outcomes.

Administrative—There are ways to be involved in the cause for social justice. You can be an activist as an individual. You also have the opportunity to engage in activism as a member of your professional nursing organization. If you take advantage of the opportunity to be an activist as a nurse, then take the time to understand the stance your profession has taken on the issue at hand. You can also take advantage of opportunities to participate in the development of your profession's stance on a given issue.

INTERNATIONAL COUNCIL OF NURSES (ICN) CODE OF ETHICS FOR NURSES

Read administratively, this view identifies the ideals set forward in the code. Find the value in the standards. How do these standards uphold the expectations for the role?

1. **Nurses and People**

   Administrative—This element of the ICN code begins with an affirmation of human rights, a fundamental concern in deontological ethics. Affirming human rights requires respect for individuals. The ICN code associates respect for individuals with the informed consent process, which is central to respect for autonomy.

2. **Nurses and Practice**

   Administrative—There are several ethical skill sets that you bring to your practice. Responsibility, personal health practices, standards of personal conduct, along with your nursing skills are all part of professional integrity. There is an expectation for the role of nursing. Promoting yourself as an exemplar of these standards brings self-worth and elevates the profession.

3. **Nurses and the Profession**

   Administrative—As you promote personal responsibility and accountability according the standards of ethical nursing practice, you also find that you are involved in determining what those standards should be. You are the profession. Your role as a nurse positions you to stand for the integrity of the profession as a whole in addition to your own integrity as a member of that profession. This means that you have a personal stake in what the standards of the profession are.

4. **Nurses and Coworkers**

   Administrative—As a professional with integrity, you accept responsibility and accountability for your ethical competency in your role. You also recognize that the standards that apply to you professionally equally apply to your colleagues in nursing and related professions. This recognition should inspire coworkers into a spirit of support and collaboration.

JAPANESE NURSING ASSOCIATION (JNA) CODE OF ETHICS

This code is presented through the lens of strategic-level thinking. A code of ethics can provide guidance for decision-making. It is not as specific as protocols, orders, or procedures, of course. The code identifies the core purpose of the profession. How does it help you to make decisions that are appropriate to that purpose?

1. **Nurses respect human life, human dignity, and human rights.**

   Strategic—Administratively, respect is an acknowledgment of rights and value. Strategically, it guides behavior. What do you have to do to demonstrate to someone that you show them respect? Respect can imply acting with manners and etiquette. What does it mean to treat someone this way? Consider cultural differences here. Pay attention to detail, as advised under the Ethical Assessment Model. What does it mean to show this person respect in this situation?

2. **Nurses provide nursing care to all people equally, regardless of their nationality, race, ethnicity, religion, faith, age, gender, sex and sexual orientation, social status, economic status, lifestyle, or the nature of their health problems.**

   Strategic—Understand what respect and acceptance mean within your professional responsibilities. Doing your job means that you know your role. You will encounter people who have attributes that will stand out to you. They will be marked, as it were, as different in some way. These differences are not what you are to attend to. The differences that should command your attention are those that are discovered in the assessment of a patient's condition. Treat the patient, whoever the patient is.

3. **Nurses build trusting relationships with people receiving care and provide nursing care based on the relationship.**

   Strategic—We will explore the importance of trust in the chapter on Advocacy. Trust involves dedication to the patient and to the role of the nurse. There are elements of being trustworthy that need to be brought into your practice.

4. **Nurses respect and protect the rights of people to information and self-determination.**

   Strategic—Respecting rights of the patient to their own information and to make decisions about their care affects health outcomes. There are policies and procedures to cover privacy, confidentiality, and consent. Beyond these policies and procedures, you can adopt concern for these as central to your professional practice.

5. **Nurses honor confidentiality and strive for the protection of personal information, while using appropriate discretion in the sharing of this information.**

   Strategic—The information you gather is not yours, it belongs to the patient. Guarding the patient's information keeps intact trust that you have built with the patient.

6. **Nurses protect and safeguard clients, when their care is inhibited or their safety is threatened.**

   Strategic—Recognize the vulnerability of your patients. Act as an advocate and promote a culture of safety.

7. **Nurses clearly recognize their own responsibility and competence and take their own responsibility for the nursing care they provide.**

   Strategic—Responsibility and accountability are more than abstract duties. They are what you do. Responsibility and accountability are in your performance. This is why you need to know your role. This is the importance of maintaining your skill.

8. **Nurses always strive to maintain and develop competence by continuous learning, as part of their own responsibility.**

   Strategic—You need to maintain and increase your level of expertise. There are requirements for continuing education. Policy dictates much of this, but the way you approach your continuing education is part of your accountability to yourself and to your profession. Education is ongoing. The practical purpose is to keep you updated in your skills and to cultivate the continual development of your ability to provide care.

9. **Nurses provide nursing care in collaboration with other nurses as well as health-care and welfare personnel.**

   Strategic—The provision of health care is a process. The process is to serve the delivery of care. Know your role in this process. Understand that other professionals contribute to the process as well. How is your role shaped by what the other professionals bring to the delivery of care?

10. **Nurses determine and implement desirable standards for nursing practice, management, education, and research, in order to provide quality nursing care.**

    Strategic—Policies and procedures and not just given. They have to be created and assessed and revised. Standards for education also have to be kept up to date to serve the needs of patients and the public. There are a variety of ways to participate in the development of procedures and educational standards.

11. **Nurses endeavor to create and develop professional knowledge and skills through research and practice, and to contribute to the progress of nursing science.**

    Strategic—You make a persistent contribution to your patients. Similarly, you can make an ongoing contribution to the advancement of knowledge in the nursing practice. Stay up to date on current research and, possibly, participate in that research. You can also assess and improve your own practice.

12. **Nurses strive to protect and promote their own physical and mental health in order to provide quality nursing care.**

    Strategic—You have to take care of yourself in order to take care of someone else. Self-care was addressed earlier in the examination of the ICN code. There, we treated it administratively. Here, as a strategic concern, we move from self-care as an ideal to considerations of self-care as a practical goal.

13. **Nurses maintain high standards of personal conduct which enhances public confidence.**

    Strategic—This is a general direction toward virtue. Professional integrity requires a basis in personal integrity. As seen with Aristotle, the search for overall integrity is built on continuing efforts to bring specific virtues into habits of behavior.

14. **Nurses share with society the responsibility for environmental issues, so that people can obtain better health.**

    Strategic—The nurse can influence health. Health doesn't just happen inside the body. We can discuss many aspects of health—mental, spiritual, and emotional. We can also identify many factors outside the body that impact health. These factors are in our social, occupational, and natural environments. For the nurse to influence health, the nurse can also find some way to attend to these environmental factors. The JNA code cites both the natural and the social environments, which pertain to issues of public health, environmental ethics, and social justice.

15. **Nurses, through the professional organization, participate in establishing a system for quality nursing care and contribute to the development of a better society.**

    Strategic—There are many ways to be involved in the work for social justice. As an individual, you have many options to become involved and many causes from which to choose. As we work for social justice, we find power and voice in gathering into organizations to bring our collective talents to bear on specific causes. As a professional, you belong to an organization that has an interest in certain causes. There is already opportunity for you to work for social justice as a member of your profession.

CANADIAN NURSES ASSOCIATION (CNA) CODE OF ETHICS

Professional integrity has a personal component. How do you see yourself as upholding the standards of the role? How can you look at the code as a personal affirmation? What can the code mean to you? Despite differences in administrative and strategic levels, how you behave at the bedside really doesn't change. How does this code help direct you there? The code positions you as a compassionate professional.

1. **Providing Safe, Compassionate, Competent, and Ethical Care**

   Interpersonal—Your professional role is to provide care. Care has many dimensions. The way you provide care depends on the unit you're on. Delivering medicines on time, helping someone to the bathroom etc. The kind of care you provide depends on the needs of the patient. The care you provide occurs within a team process. All of this demands your skill. In all of this, there is an important place for compassion. The care is not delivered of its own; it is provided by you—a human being interacting with another human being.

2. **Promoting Health and Well Being**

   Interpersonal—Compassionate awareness means paying attention to the whole patient, including determinants of health like economics, education, physical environment, social support network, genetics, health services, and gender. Providing compassionate care may require a nurse to go beyond the use of clinical skills. Nurses may need to educate patients, involve other members of the clinical team, or reach out to resources in the community. Nurses may even have to advocate for a patient who is being treated unjustly.

3. **Promoting and Respecting Informed Decision-Making**

   Interpersonal—This is the compassionate part of respecting autonomy. It's not just handing information to the patient but engaging with the patient to do one's best to make sure the information is understood. Compassion also requires the willingness to allow patients to make decisions in the manner that feels appropriate to them. This involves compassionate communication. Telling patients what they need to know in a way they need to hear it. Most importantly, this involves listening to the patients' needs and autonomous interest in directing their own lives.

4. **Honoring Dignity**

   Interpersonal—This is not just acknowledging the abstract dignity of someone who is an instance of humanity. At this level, dignity means witnessing this person as unique and significant. Each human being has a need to be recognized as someone of worth, someone who matters. Have the willingness to engage, interact, and be attentive to the person.

5. **Maintaining Privacy and Confidentiality**

   Interpersonal—Though narratives are to be told, remember that each person's narrative belongs to that person. Someone else's story does not belong to you. Someone's story is worth telling only to those who will listen and honor the trust in receiving the narrative. Be worthy of this trust.

6. **Promoting Justice**

   Interpersonal—This is a necessary component of the compassionate treatment of others. Recognize the worth of each individual. See the person; hear the voice of the person. Do not dismiss or stigmatize someone as a member of some group of others. Compassionately stand for those whose voices have been diminished or taken away. When you are faced with one whose voice has been silenced; listen closely to that person and do what you can to help that person find voice. Remember that voice isn't always spoken or written language. People can speak through tears, through gestures, through posture. Sometimes you may need to translate tears into advocacy.

7. **Being Accountable**

   Interpersonal—Compassion involves the willingness to pay attention to one who is in need. You will encounter many different people whose needs you can attend to. One person you will always be with is you. Pay attention to yourself. Understand the scope and limits of your practice. Understand what you have done well and where you need to improve. Understand your own needs for self-care. You are accountable to your employer, to your profession, and to regulatory agencies. You are also accountable to yourself. This is an authentic form of accountability.

EXERCISE

Return to the ICN, JNA, and CNA codes of ethics. Read them from the other levels of ethical assessment. (For instance, read the ICN code interpersonally or strategically.) Discuss how this reading impacts the insight you derive from the provision of this code.

For further perspective, compare and contrast these codes of ethics. What stands out to you as similarities or differences? What can you say about the culture in which each code arises?

These codes of ethics are not just *theirs* or *ours*. The spirit and the essence of these codes of ethics remains very much the same. Nursing as a profession is global. While each professional gathering will offer its own code that speaks within the perspective of a given culture, you see the spirit of nursing within all of them.

EXERCISE

From the perspective of a nurse, do you believe that each of these four codes applies to you? Can you see yourself in all of these? Discuss.

ETHICAL RELATIVISM

Ethical relativism holds that moral standards and beliefs are shaped by and relative to a number of cultural and personal factors.

Ethical relativism is built on the observation that moral standards and beliefs are shaped by many factors. Personality and personal experiences help to influence the moral beliefs of individuals. There is evidence that moral reactions can be shaped by factors such as levels of certain neurotransmitters in the brain and by negative experiences. Cultural influences likely also have some influence on personality (Triandis & Suh, 2002). Individuals within a given culture will tend to share certain beliefs that might not be shared by people in other cultures. Cultural influences like language, religious beliefs, observances, gender roles, dietary practices, art and entertainment all contribute to, and are reflected in, normative aspects of a culture such as laws and moral beliefs.

What are we to say about the influence of culture on moral beliefs once we recognize it? Perspectives here vary. Typically, ethical relativism is taken to imply a need for open-minded restraint before passing judgment about the beliefs and practices of another culture that strike us as offensive or perverse. Generally speaking, any attitude that promotes approaching moral issues with an open mind has merit because an open mind serves critical thinking.

There is also a common response to ethical relativism that calls for utter restraint in the face of cultural difference. This response holds that we must never judge another culture's beliefs no matter how offensive we find the practice to be. *They are entitled to their beliefs* is a frequently heard expression from those who hold this response. Here, there is some interest in holding an open mind, but the effect is to have an uncritical mind as well. This response also takes present cultural beliefs as somehow inherently authoritative—if it is a belief held within a culture then it must be respected. In Chapter 1, we noted that one's personal moral reactions are not necessarily what one ought to believe. The argument rested on the fact that personal moral reactions can be incomplete, can be changed, and can be improved upon. Similarly, we can see that cultural beliefs need not be regarded as unshakeable, reliable grounds for individual belief.

Cultural standards are not uniform. Moral controversies exist within cultures. Two people who share comparable demographic profiles can differ in their personalities, personal experiences, beliefs and values. Not everyone believes the same things or believe the same things with the same degree of conviction.

It is especially important to recognize the power structures that exist within societies. What outsiders might take to be a belief that is common within a culture might be a belief that is promoted by, and for the benefit of, a power elite. Such is often the case in cultures in which the oppression of a minority group (women or ethnic minorities, for example) is practiced (Okin, 1999). When this occurs, cultural structures are often such that those in oppressed groups have little voice to speak out against practices that harm them. Hence, the lack of known internal complaints against certain cultural practices is not necessarily an indication that everyone within the culture shares the beliefs that underpin those practices.

Cultural standards are not necessarily consistent. Cultural standards develop over time and from a variety of influences. At any point in time some of those beliefs might not logically fit with other beliefs. Inconsistencies like these can fuel controversies or rest at the heart of observed hypocritical behaviors. Controversies and hypocrisies, in turn, can inspire movements for change.

Cultural standards are not permanently fixed. Cultures change over time; their beliefs and practice change as well. The mechanisms of change are varied. Individuals and groups within a culture can push for change in response to controversies and new ideas. Cultural beliefs also are subject to change as the culture comes to interact with people of other cultures. People of different cultures can exchange ideas. We can learn from each other, debate and discuss with each other. When this dialogue is engaged with a critical open mind, we can find that there is much to learn. Those who support the noncritical view of relativism sometimes express concern about one culture trying to force a change of beliefs on another. Efforts to force a change in beliefs can be worrying, but changes in cultural beliefs need not be forced. If intercultural dialogue is engaged, change can happen. An essential element of such dialogue will be an open-mindedness on both sides. As long as

Tolerance is the capacity to endure something that is a source of hardship or distress. Ethically, it pertains to restraint in expressing moral judgment.

at least one side is convinced of the correctness of its beliefs, dialogue is less likely to happen.

Tolerance carries the sense of encountering something that causes one distress but is not deemed to be severe enough of a problem that it is worth prohibiting or curtailing. Tolerance appears to apply best to nuisances. When you tolerate something, you put up with it. In an ethical sense, toleration is called for when someone's behavior annoys, disturbs, or even offends you, and yet you decide not to act to address that behavior. There can be many reasons to decide not to intervene against this distressing behavior. For instance, you might believe that such an effort would cause more harm than good; that the distressing action isn't really that bad; that the source of the distress wouldn't react positively to your intervention.

Justifications of the noncritical form of ethical relativism will sometimes defend tolerance by claiming that we should not *force our views on others*. While this has merit, intervention need not—and should not—amount to forcing people to change their beliefs. As discussed, this view is problematic because of the blanket way in which moral discourse is dismissed. There are productive and reasonable ways to intervene when an act is performed in such a way as to cause us moral offense.

While tolerance is an ethically challenging idea, it has an important place in health care. In your professional capacity, your role is to care for your patient. You might find that you feel distress due to a patient's behavior, appearance, or expressed beliefs. The place of your professional interaction with this patient is not the place for you to initiate a dialogue about your moral differences. This is a place that is to be devoted to the promotion of that patient's health outcomes. Interpersonally, your task is to see past differences in culture and beliefs that distress you. Your task is to see the patient, see the person who is beyond the culture—the person who is vulnerable before you, who needs your professional skill and integrity.

None of your patients will be exactly alike. Yet, they are not so different that they are utterly alien to you. The foundation set for this text holds that harm is a foundational concept in health care ethics. We all are subject to harm. We all have an interest in avoiding needless harm and in alleviating the harm we suffer. Recognize the individuality in your patient. Recognize also that each patient is vulnerable, desires not to suffer, and is in need of your competent and compassionate care. Recognize that, at least as far as health care is concerned, "We are more alike, my friends, than we are unalike" (Angelou, 1997).

One other concern about noncritical ethical relativism should be raised: It can inspire a view that people of different cultures are alone in setting and living up to their own moral standards. When we recognize that individuals differ in their moral beliefs, a sense of isolation can develop. We can begin to develop the notion that we are left to our own devices to figure out how to embrace and cultivate integrity (however we describe integrity). This is not at all the case. The professional oaths and the codes of ethics are meant to offer aid in envisioning what it is like to live with professional integrity. There is something else that can help as well. This is a form of dialogue conveyed through a role model.

ROLE MODELS

The initial work to develop integrity is a matter of identifying target virtues and finding a way to emulate them in your own activity. Like learning to play a musical instrument, you really learn virtue by practicing with someone, getting feedback, seeing the interaction. We need to practice virtuous acts in order to become virtuous. As we practice, we develop habits of acting virtuously. As we develop these habits, we position ourselves to genuinely develop these virtues.

It is one thing to be told what virtues to develop. It is another to have someone else who personally embodies some of these virtues. Someone who mentors you. Someone you can watch or envision and, in observing this person, you can begin to figure out what it might be to act virtuously in this way. You can then begin to model your own actions after the example of this person. Habits can develop from there. Virtue can mature. Such an exemplar is a **role model**.

Role models can have appeal and influence on all three levels of ethical assessment. On the interpersonal level, a role model is someone who stands out to you, who connects with you, as an exemplar of integrity. Your role model needs to be realistic enough and relatable enough for you to imagine yourself in that person's place, acting as that person does.

On the strategic level, the role model exemplifies virtuous conduct. Your role model reveals enough about virtuous behavior to provide you with lessons. Where you encounter frustrations in your profession or in your own behavior, your role model can offer suggestions—either in the form of advice or in the form of example.

On an administrative level, a role model points toward an ideal. The role model need not be perfect. You don't have to see full integrity in the person of your role model. But, through your role model, you should be able to get a clearer glimpse of what the ideal is like. More to the point, your role model should show you the real possibility of personal growth through devotion to moving toward this ideal.

A **role model** is someone who is accepted as a person who presents an example worth imitating in one's own behavior.

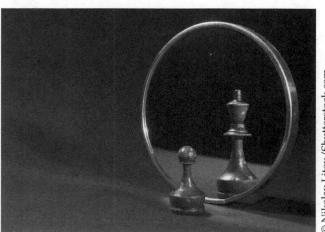

© Nikolay Litov/Shutterstock.com

Figure 4.3 A role model can help us see our potential to become more than what we are

A role model isn't necessarily someone who says "Be like me". This is a person of integrity. This integrity might include humility that prevents the role model from this sort of self-promotion. The leadership of the role model is evident more in the way this person goes about fulfilling the professional role and through the character that shines out in the performance of that role's tasks.

Professions may have real or legendary role models. In nursing, the classic role model is Florence Nightingale. Florence Nightingale is the professional ideal of what a nurse should be. She believed that morality came from within the person and ethics addressed the wholeness for providing care.

Florence Nightingale was born in 1820. In her teens, she determined to pursue a career in nursing despite the objections of her parents. At the time, nursing had a poor reputation, seen as menial labor. In 1844, she enrolled in a school for nurses. Ten years later, during the Crimean War, Nightingale was called upon to assemble a team of nurses to attend to wounded British soldiers. Appalled by the unsanitary conditions of the military hospital, Nightingale undertook the task of reforming sanitation and nursing practice. She was known to check on soldiers at night, carrying a lamp to light her way.

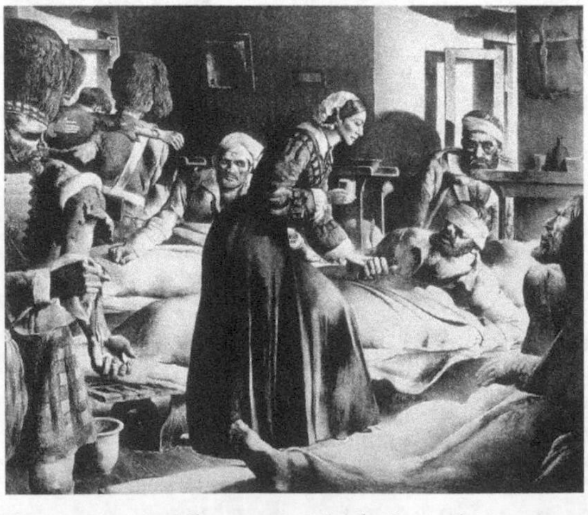

Nightingale became known as the *Lady of the Lamp*. Her dedication to her patients, her efforts to reform nursing, and her devotion to her profession stood out. The figure of Nightingale carrying the lamp came to symbolize her integrity as a nurse. In this image and in the standards and writings she left behind, we have a role model.

© Everett Historical/Shutterstock.com

Figure 4.4 Florence Nightingale caring for soldiers during the Crimean War

When it comes to integrity, if you're just taught obedience and the letter of the policies you are to comply with, then you're not yet doing ethics. Ethics involves critical thinking, taking on perspectives, seeking understanding. Integrity is more than just doing what's expected. It also involves the effort to understand why it makes sense to do these things. In the same way, we can do better than simply accept Florence Nightingale as the image of a nurse. What can we learn by examining professional nursing through her example, her writings, and her influence?

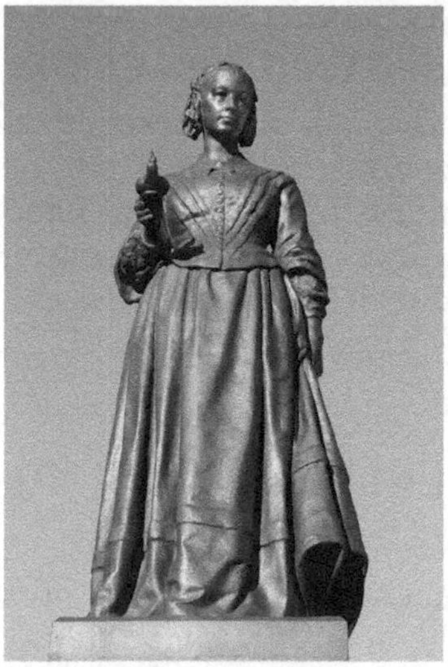

TAKEAWAY

As a student you might be enthusiastic about going into the profession. You might desire to be on your own as a health-care professional. At the same time, as everything is new, you can feel insecure, even a little intimidated. At the cusp of a professional career, you might wonder what this life will be like. Your role models, code of ethics, and efforts to cultivate virtue won't tell you what your life as

© Tony Baggett/Shutterstock.com

Figure 4.5 A statue of Florence Nightingale in Waterloo Place, Westminster, London, UK

a professional will be, but they will all be part of what you can draw from to guide you into your future. As your career continues, these tools of professional integrity can follow you and serve as continual reminders to help freshen you in your practice to remind you of what your service is about.

CASE STUDIES

CASE STUDY 4.1—FLORENCE NIGHTINGALE

Research and describe Florence Nightingale's work in the Crimean War. Describe her actions through the Ethical Assessment Model. Next, select one of the nursing codes of ethics described above. Explain which of the provisions of that code are illustrated by Nightingale's actions. Do you see any discrepancy between Nightingale's actions and the code that you investigated? What does this say about changes in the professional role of nurses?

CASE STUDY 4.2—ETHICAL ASSESSMENT AND CODES OF ETHICS

Find a code of ethics from another allied health profession. Engage the exercise used above for the ANA Code of Ethics and interpret the provisions of the code from the administrative, strategic, and interpersonal levels of ethical assessment. Compare your findings with the nursing codes explored in this chapter. What important similarities and differences do you see?

(Continued)

CASE STUDY 4.3—CODES AND CODES AND CODES
Find a code of ethics from a profession outside of healthcare. Engage the exercise used above for the ANA Code of Ethics and interpret the provisions of the code from the administrative, strategic, and interpersonal levels of ethical assessment. Compare your findings with the nursing codes explored in this chapter. What important similarities and differences do you see?

REFERENCES

Angelou, M. (1997). *Human family*. In *I shall not be moved*. New York: Random House.

APTA. (2013). *Code of ethics for the physical therapist*. Alexandria, VA: American Physical Therapy Association. Retrieved from https://www.apta.org/uploadedFiles/APTAorg/About_Us/Policies/Ethics/CodeofEthics.pdf

Aristotle. (2002). *Nicomachean ethics* (J. Sachs, Trans.). Newbury, MA: Focus Pub./R. Pullins.

Becker, H. S. (1962). The nature of a profession. In N. B. Henry (Ed.). *Education for the professions* (pp. 24–46). Chicago: University of Chicago Press.

de Tornyay, R. (1989). The international pledge for nurses. *Journal of Nursing Education, 28*(4), 149–149.

Lasagna, L. (1964, June 28). Would Hippocrates rewrite his oath? *New York Times Magazine*. Retrieved from https://www.nytimes.com/1964/06/28/would-hippocrates-rewrite-his-oath-after-2000-years-the-greek-pledge-traditionally-taken-by-doctors-is-falling-into-disuse-a-pro.html

McBurney, B. H., & Filoromo, T. (1994). The nightingale pledge: 100 years later. *Nursing Management, 25*(2), 72.

Okin, S. M. (1999). *Is multiculturalism bad for women?* Princeton, NJ: Princeton University Press.

Triandis, H. C., & Suh, E. M. (2002). *Cultural influences on personality. Annual Review of Psychology, 53*(1), 133–160.

White, J., Phakoe, M., and Rispel, L. C. (2015) 'Practice what you preach': Nurses' perspectives on the code of ethics and service pledge in five South African hospitals. *Global Health Action 8*(1), 26341.

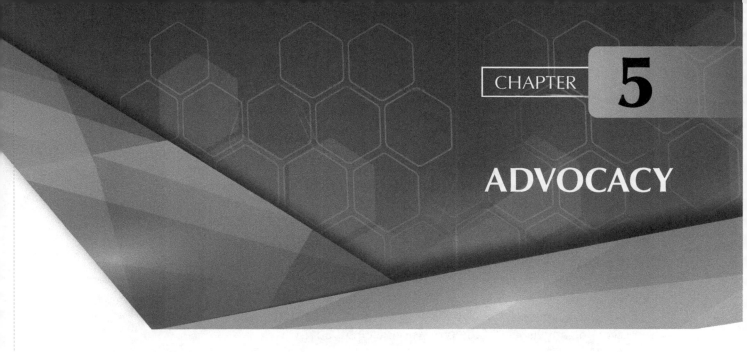

CHAPTER 5

ADVOCACY

OBJECTIVES

After completing this chapter, you will be able to . . .

1. Understand the beneficial attributes displayed in advocacy.

2. Identify the nature of trust; discuss what it means to be trustworthy.

3. Articulate veracity as a virtue and as an ethical obligation.

4. Discuss the relationship between privacy and confidentiality. Articulate the ethical significance of each.

5. Identify the expectations for fidelity and discuss the how they apply in practice.

6. Discuss how the features of advocacy apply to demonstrating respect for autonomy.

7. Apply the Ethical Assessment Model to chapter exercises and to real-life scenarios.

KEY TERMS

- Adversary
- Advocacy
- Anticipation
- Confidentiality
- Expectation
- Fidelity
- Privacy
- Trust
- Trustworthiness
- Veracity
- Vulnerability

Box 5.1

The radiologic technologist respects confidences entrusted in the course of professional practice, respects the patient's right to privacy, and reveals confidential information only as required by law or to protect the welfare of the individual or the community (ARRT, 2017).

Box 5.2 Principle of Ethics III

Individuals shall honor their responsibility to the public when advocating for the unmet communication and swallowing needs of the public and shall provide accurate information involving any aspect of the professions (ASHA, 2016).

INTRODUCTION

A patient enters a hospital in search of the best outcome. Once admitted, the patient wears a formless gown and an ID bracelet with a bar code. The patient is in a generic room with little of the familiarity and comfort of home. Illness disrupts a person's sense of normalcy (Canguilhem, 2012). This can lead to a need in the patient to be affirmed as a person who matters. The patient may yearn for some recognition as being more than a medical problem to be solved. The medical team, of course, is there precisely to identify and address the medical problem for this patient and for many others besides. There isn't time to give every patient the attention he or she might crave.

Illness and injury can alter patients' sense of normalcy. Admission to a hospital can lead to further separation from their personal sense of identity. In nursing and allied health, we have a choice; our patients don't. Patients are often looking for interpersonal connection that helps give substance to their sense of identity and affirms their worth as persons. They are willing to find this connection with the professional who is there with them at the moment—a nurse, nursing assistant, a physical therapist, a radiology tech, or anyone who looks like a competent professional.

Patients want to trust that their nurses and allied health professionals will be loyal to them. They have expectations for the care they will receive and for the way in which this care will be delivered. While some of these expectations might not be realizable, there are ethical expectations that the patient should be able to have of health-care professionals. Professional obligations and nursing duties can serve to help keep the nurse loyal to both patient and organization. In this chapter, loyalty, trust, and other traits will be explored as they pertain to patient advocacy.

ADVOCACY AND SUPPORT

Nurses and those in allied health interact with patients that span the spectrum from healthy, to sick, and to dying. The responsibilities of ethical treatment do not waver.

Nurses and allied health professionals need to be accountable for the care they provide. The pioneering model for nursing was established by Florence Nightingale. Her recommendations encouraged behaviors embodied in the integrity of the profession. The essential attribute of professional integrity is providing safe care and patient advocacy. When you show up for work you are advocating for your patients. Everyone involved with patient care should be an advocate.

Patient advocacy doesn't mean charging through the halls on a horse ready to do battle. When people say *I'm advocating for my patient,* they often use the declaration defensively. *You're not doing what I think should be done,* or, *No one is listening to me.* It's a perception of loss of value, or it's a claim that *I know the right thing to do.*

"I'm advocating for my patient!" points out what *you're* doing. We establish policies and procedures to protect the patient. We respect autonomy. If people are fulfilling their roles, then everything is geared toward advocating for the patient. True **advocacy** is a response to a call for help. It is the response to a call to come to the aid of a patient—whether the patient makes the call or it comes from someone else.

Think of a call light as an extension of the patient's voice. When the call light goes on, you respond by going into the room. Advocacy begins here. Going into the room, you find more of the patient's voice: the reason why they have put the light on. Sometimes, the reason they cite isn't the need they seek to satisfy (emotional needs, such as fright or loneliness). Do you have the willingness to identify the real need behind the call and compassionately respond?

The two words, voice and advocacy, share the same root in Latin, *voc.* Someone who needs an advocate calls for aid. To call for aid, of course, involves using one's voice. When you are being an advocate, you are projecting someone's voice. Whose voice is coming through in your advocacy? Is it your patient's? Or, is it your own?

The advocate is one who raises a voice on behalf of the one who needs aid. The core notion of advocacy is voice. Voices call out and are heard. Advocacy must involve both. If the patient can't speak, your advocacy puts you in the position of speaking on the patient's behalf. If the patient speaks—or someone speaks for the patient—that call for aid needs a response.

A patient talks to you, wanting to share some aspect of the patient's life. The patient wants to be regarded as a person. This is a call for aid. The aid you are being asked to give is acknowledgment of the patient as a person. Of course, you already know that this is a person. But you don't know *this* person—the person that the patient feels (fears) is lost. The desired narrative path for patients is a path of restitution to health

Advocacy is the act of speaking for and supporting someone in need.

(Frank, 2013). Illness or injury takes the patient out of normal life, and it is this life that the patient yearns to have given back. Talking about this normal life that the patient has been distanced from—and having this life affirmed by an attentive audience—helps connect the patient with the memory and hope of the restoration of that life.

When patients are in need of health care, there is a call for aid. When you advocate, there is value recognized in the patient. Your goal will be to support the value that is individual to the patient. Identify the value and you can identify what you are advocating. What you value is demonstrated by your actions.

Patients sometimes don't want to be helped. *Leave me alone.* They have a baseline for coping. Advocacy can mean recognizing their need at that time. Advocacy doesn't always mean doing; first, it means awareness.

Advocacy also requires technical readiness. Staying competent in your professional skills contributes to advocacy because you are prepared. Obtaining a Cardiopulmonary Resuscitation (CPR) card may seem trivial but this is one of the basic expectations for the occupation. Having achieved this basic knowledge your advocacy for a patient is demonstrated as your patients can be confident you can perform CPR if they were to need resuscitation.

It can feel like there is a disharmony in advocacy. If you feel that you are charging down the hallway on a horse proclaiming yourself as an advocate, there may be some conflict that is in need of deeper examination. The whole of health care is set up to advocate for the patient. Do you feel conflict? If so, use the Ethical Assessment Model to ask yourself if your personal moral beliefs and professional ethical standards are at odds or if they are aligned. Is there a compelling argument for your advocacy or is there an explanation for why circumstances are not as you expect them to be? Recognize the value of the patient for whom you advocate and the balance between everyone's expectations. Advocacy means meeting expectations within the profession. But everyone in the health-care team has different roles in how they are able to meet those expectations.

An **expectation** is a belief that something should happen.

The preceding exercise is a good introduction to advocating for a patient while understanding how important it is to follow orders. These are the **expectations**. This could be a dilemma, but there are choices that could resolve the issue. The nurse understands the obligation to follow orders. The nurse understands that when a patient agrees to medical care that there are expectations the patient agrees to follow also. If the patient refuses to follow, it is the patient's right. The nurse advocates for the patient and follows the doctor's orders. There is an expectation that you provide care. The doctor's orders direct you to provide care. Following these orders is a form of advocacy.

You may perceive things differently when you are alongside the patient. At the bedside you can gain insightful perspective into a patient's experiences and expectations. This is the essence of the interpersonal connection.

A patient wants to stay one more day in the hospital but the surgeon just wrote the orders to discharge the patient. The patient has confided in you that staying one more day in the hospital could help the patient feel more confident about going home. Discuss (or role play) this scenario from the perspectives of the patient and a nurse or allied health professional in whom the patient confides. Apply the Ethical Assessment Model as you explore this scenario.

Advocacy means meeting expectations. As a nurse or allied health professional, you are not in position to make choices for your patient. Your role is to meet the expectations of care. These expectations are placed by the patient or by the patient's surrogate. The expectations for treatment are set by doctors, physician assistants, or through protocol. These expectations are fundamental to health care. Let's explore what advocacy fully entails.

MORAL SAFETY NET

Patient advocacy can be seen as taking the role of a moral safety net. Make sure that the patient does not come to harm. This can provide a perspective to help members of the medical team locate themselves in a given scenario.

Safety nets are placed. For a trapeze artist, the net is placed right under where the artist is performing. That is directly between the artist and what might cause her the most harm—the ground. As a patient's safety net, you are placed where the patient is at risk of coming to harm. You are the embodiment of the directive to at least do no harm. Your task is to position yourself with an awareness of where the activity is, where harm might arise.

Your role places you in position to help keep your patient from harm. Being in this position entails an important trust. Your patient is vulnerable; you are there to care for this

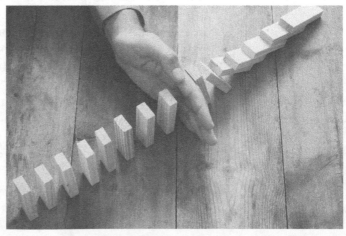

Figure 5.1

person. A net can be placed, but a professional has more to offer than the placement of the role. The net spans a performance area, and yet the net does not perform. The professional performs. The professional is aware, acts and responds. The professional with integrity brings a moral quality to the expectations held out by vulnerable patients.

It seems that there is little use in simply asking people to advocate for patients. As we've noted, the competent performance of your job is a form of advocacy. Probably, this is the form of advocacy that is most needed from you. Still, we also understand that *do your job* doesn't always capture the moral demands of your professional life. Too, "do your job" can come across as scolding or a put-down, leading to defensive declarations like, *I'm advocating for my patient!*

When we hold advocacy as an aspiration, we offer it as a virtue. Yes, it means doing your job, but we also see a quality to advocacy—a *thisness* that sets it apart from "just" doing your job. Being an advocate is not just what we are told to do; it it what we wish to be. Patient advocacy is Florence Nightingale, the Lady with the Lamp, checking on soldiers in camp at night during the Crimean War. Like most virtues, we can't give specific directions to become an advocate. There is no algorithm. We can, however, keep the levels of ethical assessment in mind and offer five elements of advocacy: Trust, Veracity, Privacy, Confidentiality, and Fidelity.

TRUST

For 16 consecutive years, Gallup polls have found that Americans have rated nurses as the professionals they trust the most (Brenan, 2017). Think of the public expectation. They imagine (or recall) encounters with nurses. They envision meeting nurses when they are in a position of need. There is an expectation that nurses will act for their best interests and will do so at both the strategic (delivering care) and interpersonal (doing so with compassion) levels. At the bottom of the Gallup poll are lobbyists and car salespeople—people who are stereotypically described as motivated by their own self-interest, possibly at the expense of the public. Where there is little trust in lobbyists, there is considerable trust in nurses. When you are vulnerable, when your resources are limited, the delivery of compassion won't threaten you.

Mayer, Davis, and Schoorman define **trust** as "the willingness of a party to be vulnerable to the actions of another party based on the expectation that the other will perform a particular action important to the trustor, irrespective of the ability to monitor or control that other party" (Mayer, Davis, & Schoorman, 1995). In advocacy, there is a commitment, a willingness, to meet the expectations of patients and of orders for patient care. Effective advocacy depends on being trustworthy.

Trust is an expectation that another has the skills of being trustworthy. Trust is having the belief that someone will assume responsibility and meet expectations.

Trustworthiness is the virtue exhibited by a medical professional that helps to inspire trust in someone else, such as a patient, a member of the patient's family, or a colleague. How does one inspire trust? That is, what is involved in being trustworthy? To explore trustworthiness, it can help to consider advocacy as the patient's call for aid. Calling for aid comes from a position of vulnerability. The patient needs aid and also feels exposed. Trust is an expectation of safety.

Imagine being in a position of extreme vulnerability. You cannot see to your own most desperate need. You cannot protect yourself.

Alvaro is in the neurological ICU after experiencing a stroke. Until this catastrophic event, Alvaro had no known health problems. Like most people who do not know the trials of chronic or intense medical problems, Alvaro had taken his health for granted. Now, he feels weak and experiences paralysis in one arm and leg. Because this arm is the one that he uses to write, the paralysis adds to his frustration. He is aphasic and is frustrated by his inability to communicate. He doesn't feel like himself and fears that he could lose more of his mind or body at any moment. Alvaro feels utterly helpless. He finds that he relies on his nurses, nursing assistants, and visiting family members for everything.

Alvaro's case is one of utter vulnerability. His ability to see to his own care is diminished. His ability to move is seriously compromised. He is experiencing anxiety. Moreover, he cannot communicate any of this. What he knows is that he is dependent. He feels that he is a burden—a burden to be carried, protected, and tended. From his nurses and nursing assistants, he calls out for aid in terms of the skills they can provide. More, he calls out for these skills to be offered when needed. Since his needs are pervasive—and somewhat unpredictable, in the case of his fears of another event—he calls out for these skills to be available when he needs them. That is, he calls out for reliability.

To be effective, clinical skills need to be sustainable. Clinical settings are designed to ensure care that is reliably available. Clinical systems are designed to foster trust. One way in which trust is fostered is by assigning roles and responsibility. This is done at the administrative and strategic levels (Peter & Morgan, 2001).

In a trusting relationship, we each accept responsibility toward each other and believe that the other will live up to responsibility. Trustworthiness is part of your skill set. It is part of ethical competency. When ethics is applied to trust, it assures that deviations are least likely to happen. The expectations of duty are upheld (Rutherford, 2014).

There is an expectation when trust is involved. There is an expectation that the person you trust will be reliable. How do you know? First, you trust someone based on the role that person has toward you or based on rules that regulate how someone is to act toward you. This person is anticipated to be worthy of trust on the basis of an administrative-level judgment that this person can be categorized into a certain role. Over time as someone acts to meet your expectations and does so reliably, this

Trustworthiness is the skill set that demonstrates that one will strive to live up to the expectations of those who place trust and take all care to avoid causing them harm.

person has demonstrated being worthy of trust through the use of skills. This establishes trust at the strategic level. Further, and deeper, demonstrations of trust come from those who approach you with compassion, who show the willingness to respond to you in your vulnerability.

Return to our example of Alvaro. A person he has never seen before walks into his room and says, "Hi, I'm Ruby. I'm your nurse for today." Alvaro trusts Ruby because she has the role of someone who can care for him and help him. This is trust at the administrative level. Ruby fits a category that Alvaro regards as worthy of his trust.

The next day, Ruby has Alvaro as a patient again. Alvaro trusts her because she provided him with good and reliable care yesterday. This is trust at the strategic level. Alvaro has some evidence that he can rely on Ruby's care.

Alvaro feels that he is at risk. His condition makes him so. While he has few resources, he tries to protect himself to the extent that he is able. He withholds his emotions. Of the people on his medical team, only Ruby has gained his trust such that Alvaro will let down his defenses enough to let her know the sorrow and fear he keeps inside. This is trust at the interpersonal level. Alvaro feels that Ruby recognizes his suffering and acknowledges him for who he is.

To be trustworthy in working with a patient, you need to combine technical skill and compliance with policy and procedure. There also needs to be competence at the interpersonal level. Patients want and need you to be skilled at the technical aspects of your job. This shows that you are good at caring for them. They also want to feel that you care about them.

Vulnerability is the state of being exposed to harm and to risk of further harm.

Trust is conditional. As it rests on responding to someone in their **vulnerability**, so trust itself is vulnerable. The risk to trust is that the one trusted might not meet the expectations of the one who offers trust. It can be lost.

Trust is not anything that can be given upon command. You can demonstrate your trustworthiness by obtaining your license or by demonstrating your skills through the performance of your job. And yet, you might have a patient who withholds trust.

Anticipation describes an attitude in which one prepares for a possible event to occur.

Anticipation and expectation both orient toward future events. Expectation differs from anticipation relative to confidence and need. If you are certain that a given event will occur, you expect it. If you are fairly confident that it will occur, though you admit that it might not, then you anticipate it. If you look forward to the meeting of a pressing need—like a nurse bringing your pain medication—then you expect this. If you look forward to something that is welcome but not quite needed, you might anticipate it.

As noted, you will face the expectations held by your patient. You will also face the expectations represented in your orders for treatment. It might also be the case that your expectations for what the patient needs won't neatly align with the expectations that the patient actually holds for desired care. Ideally, the skilled care you give will please your patient. Your professional integrity should direct you to be trustworthy. However, even if you are trustworthy, you will not always be trusted. This is important to keep in mind. Compassion is often reciprocated. Compassionate care often elicits trust, but there are times where the reward for your compassionate care is the self-satisfaction that you have been worthy of trust—even if that trust was not forthcoming.

Trustworthiness is responsibility and accountability. Responsibility is an internal motivation to act. It is your own assessment of how you should act with integrity. Accountability is an external motivation because poor choices can be sanctioned and good choices can be rewarded.

Trustworthiness is a skill. As an ethical skill, we can treat it as a virtue. This is a skill pertaining to the professional–patient relationship. We can further explore this relationship and trustworthiness, by examining four other relevant concepts.

EXERCISE

Can we explain all four of Beauchamp and Childress' principles in terms of trust? For instance, we could describe nonmaleficence as having trust that someone will not cause needless harm. Try this for beneficence, autonomy, and justice. Discuss the insights you derive from this exercise.

PRINCIPLES AND ADVOCACY

In *Principles of Biomedical Ethics*, Beauchamp and Childress examine four aspects of the patient–professional relationship: Veracity, Privacy, Confidentiality, and Fidelity. These are offered as *rules*, distinct from the four main principles that occupy much of the text. Beauchamp and Childress distinguish principles from rules. Both guide behavior in deontological fashion, but principles are described as more general than rules. Because of their comparative specificity, rules have a narrower scope than do principles. Thus, Beauchamp and Childress offer their four principles for the whole of biomedical ethics while these four rules find applicability within the patient–professional relationship (Beauchamp & Childress, 2013, p. 14).

VERACITY

Veracity is the responsibility to provide accurate and objective information.

Veracity is an interest in truth. This is not a blanket rule of being open and honest in all situations about all things. Specific to the patient–professional relationship, veracity is the expectation that patients be informed about their conditions and treatments in a timely and accurate manner. The delivery of content should be sensitive to the patient's capacity to understand.

Truth-telling keeps a patient informed, involves the patient in decision-making, and contributes to a trusting relationship. It has strategic value. Telling a patient the truth also has administrative value insofar as it can be can be seen as a respect for the patient as a human being, facilitating the patient's autonomous participation in decision-making about treatment options. Truth-telling also aligns with interpersonal connection as it fosters a trusting relationship between professional and patient.

Veracity has a dual purpose: safety and patient autonomy. Respecting patient autonomy can be interpreted culturally. But whoever makes decisions for the patient still needs to be told the truth.

EXERCISE

Elroy is an echocardiogram technician. He is in a room in the ICU performing an echocardiogram on Marilyn, a sedated and intubated 82-year-old female patient. Also in the room are Marilyn's overly involved husband and two daughters. As Elroy is performing the echocardiogram, Marilyn's family members are asking Elroy to tell them what he sees. "What does this mean? What does it show?" they ask. Use the Ethical Assessment Model to determine how should Elroy respond. Explain how Elroy's response respects veracity.

Ideally, truth-telling can enhance health outcomes (Stewart, 1995). Patients who are informed tend to trust their medical team more. As trust and information improves, so does patient compliance (Eraker, Kirscht, & Becker, 1984). Patients who are better informed about their treatment and conditions may experience less distress from their treatment. When truth-telling leads to better outcomes or better patient satisfaction (Kaplan, Greenfield, Gandek, Rogers, & Ware,

1996), the rule seems straightforward. Tell the truth: Help patients understand and comply with their treatment. As you doubtless expect, veracity is not always so easy.

Patients or family members will often reach out to those they trust—nurses or allied health professionals—and give voice to their fears. *What's going to happen to me? Do you think he's going to make it? What do you see on the ultrasound?*

Remember your role. It's not your place to offer a diagnosis or a prognosis. You don't know the future. You also don't know what the person who asks the question has in mind. However, in asking you a question like this, the person is reaching out to you for a response. Respond to the person. Have the willingness to look through this awkward situation and face the person who has asked this uncomfortable question.

Above all, don't evade the question. If you pass off the question or resort to a trite answer (*Everything's going to be just fine!*) it can very well come across as passing off the person who asked the question. Your honest response is a demonstration of respect for the person.

Tell the truth but be mindful of how you tell it. Respect the person. Respect your role and recognize that your role is suited to advocacy. Your role will help you to understand what you may say. If your only truthful answer is "I don't know," then say as much. Whatever you say, there is now the matter of *how* you say it. Have the willingness to respect the person, and to regard this person as someone who matters. Be willing to talk to this person.

PRIVACY

There is a basic need to feel that we belong with other people, to feel that we are significant because these people regard us as such. To be regarded as significant also entails an element of respect. This means respect for your individuality. You are significant because you can connect with other people, but also because you are you—irreplaceable and unrepeatable. There is an element of mystery to each unique human being. As we seek to belong, so we also feel a need to protect some of what makes us individual. The right for **privacy** is an extension of a need to keep some elements of oneself closed from public view. The central component of privacy, then, is access.

Protecting privacy is part of respect for patient autonomy. Patients have interests in determining who has access to certain information about them. Restricting access to information is a matter of self-determination. Self-determination is a process by which people exercise control over their own lives. Managing personal information is part of that process.

Privacy is an individual's right to determine who has access to certain information about that individual.

Think about what kinds of information patients might want to keep private and why. How do you protect privacy interests? How does the Ethical Assessment Model help to identify issues of privacy? What policies and procedures apply to privacy?

There are steps you take to ensure privacy. These are steps taken to control who has access to information about your patient. There are policies and procedures to protect the privacy of patient records. Think about all the other ways in which access to information about the patient can be controlled. Close a door. Draw a curtain. The patient is not always able to enact these protections. Your help is needed in order to protect and bolster the patient's privacy.

Violations of privacy are described as invasions. Invaders enter into areas where they are unwelcome. The imagery is suggestive. Invaders not only intrude, they stake a claim: *This is mine now.* Those who invade privacy don't necessarily claim information for their own, but they assume a right to access that which has not been granted. This assumption can be injurious to the one whose privacy has been invaded.

CONFIDENTIALITY

Confidentiality is an obligation not to disclose information given without express permission from the source of that information.

Confidentiality is a special duty following from the right to privacy. Privacy is a door. This door can be closed to certain individuals and opened to others. Respecting a patient's right to privacy means giving the patient the authority to determine who may pass through the door and who may not. Confidentiality is an expectation for those people who pass through the door. Now that you have access to the patient's private information, what do you do with it?

Confidentiality is tightly regulated. Information is a gateway to someone's being. Exposing information reveals aspects of the person that the person might not wish to be viewed by others. Exposing information without the person's consent is a violation of autonomy. Administratively, protecting confidentiality demonstrates respect for a patient's rights.

See how closely we align information about a person with personhood itself. We respect autonomy through the consent process by providing the patient with information and seeking specific information from the patient—namely, consent for a procedure. As we offer care for a patient, we pledge respect for the patient by protecting access to the patient's information and to keep that information confidential.

We treat information as an extension of the patient. Private information is the person extended throughout the sphere of her or his life. The information about that person can let you see into the person's past medical history. Information could enable you to see private social interactions, economic status, and habits, a history of decisions and personal preferences, a history perhaps of accomplishments and mistakes. Access to information means access to the person.

EXERCISE

Describe a situation that impacts on privacy and confidentiality. Explain the difference between privacy and confidentiality in the scenario you've created. Use the Ethical Assessment to help determine any possible difference between respecting privacy and respecting confidentiality.

FIDELITY

Another way to look at advocacy is to take note of its opposite. The opposite of being an advocate is being an **adversary**. An adversary is an opponent. Where an advocate will speak for the patient and respond to the patient's call for aid, an adversary will be a reason why the patient continues to call for aid.

The adversary will violate nonmaleficence or beneficence. An opponent can create harm where it didn't previously exist. An opponent can also withhold benefit that could be offered. An opponent can ignore a call for aid or silence the voice that would call out. An adversary needn't have the intent to cause harm. Opposition can occur through a lack of devotion.

> An **adversary** is an opponent. Ethically, this is someone who needlessly causes harm or interferes with efforts to grow.

FIDELITY IS DEVOTION

Devotion means to set something apart, to hold it in such regard that you will keep attention fixed on it. Devotion responds to what you value, to what you hold as important. Where there is devotion there is a feeling of a need for your attention and action. There is commitment and responsibility. Fidelity in your professional integrity is twofold. Your devoted commitment is to your patients and to your practice.

We often associate devotion with love, with passion, and with instinctual feelings. Indeed, devotion can be felt—as through empathy—fitting with one's moral reactions. In this way, devotion is more of an expression of what you feel. The way you see the world motivates how you act in it. See the world through your empathy and you see it in a biased way. You are not consciously seeking to be adversarial, but bias could lead you to miss something important. If you see the world only through your feelings, you might actually overlook something important about the patient or profession to which you are to be devoted.

You feel mirrored suffering in empathy. You feel motivation and you need to do something with this. You recognize that your discomfort is initiated by the suffering of your patient. But your reaction is a reaction to the suffering that *you* feel. You are representing your sense that you have to do something with your suffering. Proclaiming your advocacy is one way of doing something. But the suffering you're trying to address might be your own discomfort. Compassion is a better ground for devotion. The willingness to identify the patient—and not your own suffering—as an object of devotion is essential to providing effective care.

Devotion isn't valuable just as something to have. Devotion has to have an object, a devotion *to* something. It is meaningless to talk about being devoted without some reference to what one is devoted to. This is to say that devotion alone cannot be considered a virtue or a duty. Devotion only becomes a virtue when you recognize a duty or expectation to respond to someone or something with loyalty. To be devoted to something is to hold it as having a special value that requires you to regard it as taking some priority over other concerns.

It can be useful to think of devotion in terms of making and keeping promises. When a patient enters into your care, there is an assumed promise made that you will give some priority to this patient's care. More broadly, your professional oath is a form of promise. In taking this oath, you make a pledge to set professional integrity as a priority. In other words, **fidelity** means being aware of your professional priorities and using those priorities as a guide for your actions.

Fidelity is devotion to a person or cause, characterized by loyalty and advocacy.

You will notice a similarity in the words *fidelity* and *fiduciary*. Both words extend from a common root in Latin. Fidelity comes from *fidelis*, meaning *faith*. *Fiduciary* comes from *fidere*, meaning *to trust*. The patient needs medical treatment. As a consequence of this need, the patient has a further need to trust that members of the medical team will exercise their skills and expertise for the best interests of the patient.

Devotion extends from the fiduciary nature of the relationship between a patient and a health-care professional. The patient is rendered vulnerable due to disease, injury, or disability. The professional offers service and expertise that the patient needs. By nature of this relationship, patients must be able to trust that their health-care professionals will take their needs seriously and care for them.

Nurses are prone to feeling conflicts where fidelity is concerned (Beauchamp & Childress, 2013, pp. 327). People can have different expectations when it comes to a patient's care. The perspectives of the patient, members of the patient's family, the physician and other members of the health-care team all have their perspectives. Due to these different perspectives, expectations can vary and sometimes come into conflict.

Be careful not to simply react to your perception of conflict. The appearance of conflict can narrow our vision. We can initially believe that we have to choose between this position or that position—between the patient or the physician, for instance. Facing that choice means facing a choice between two objects of fidelity—between a promise to advocate for the patient and a promise to professional integrity. When you perceive such conflict and fear that you are faced with such a choice, pause and perform your ethical analysis.

Not all disagreements about patient care are ethical disagreements. The Ethical Assessment Model can help build perspective. As you identify the background, you'll take note of the different people in the situation and their expectations. Focus on this as you assess the level strategically. What information is available about the case and about the people who are setting these expectations? Understand the situation and pay attention to the people. Administratively, are there any rights being violated? What do we see if we view the issue from the standpoint of autonomy, beneficence, nonmaleficence, and justice? Strategically, how are all parties striving to promote the best outcomes? Interpersonally, are you still in position to provide compassionate care? What are the expectations of all parties involved in the conflict? Can you see the value that they find in these expectations?

AUTONOMY AND ADVOCACY

Advocacy for your patient means being trustworthy. It means adhering to veracity in communicating with your patient. It means protecting your patient's privacy and maintaining the trust of confidentiality. It means devotion within the scope of your practice to your patient's well-being. Advocacy means respecting the person and honoring your patient's autonomy.

In all of these aspects of advocacy, it can be said that you align with your patient. You take your patients' interests as your own. When you take an interest in your patient's autonomy, you are placing yourself in position to support the patient's right to self-determination. A patient who practices self-determination will make personal choices that are the patient's own. Just as you protect the patient's privacy, so you also honor the patient's ownership of personal choice. Thus, aligning with the patient needn't mean that you agree with every choice that your patient makes.

There will be times when your advocacy will not feel resolved. Perhaps, you see that a decision needs to be made, and you're not in position to make it. This strategic level is out of your control; outside of your role. Nursing and allied health professionals sometimes can't be heard. Strategic decisions about patient treatment are made by patients, their surrogates, and the doctors. Nurses and allied health professionals aren't consulted. This isn't your role. Your role is not to make the decision on behalf of the patient. The decision belongs to the patient.

It can be hard to watch people make decisions that you don't agree with. Keep in mind that patients make decisions based on their own perspective. Your view of a choice a patient is making is not the same view that the patient has. To align with the patient's right to choose means acknowledging that patient has a way of viewing this situation that may be, to some degree, a mystery to you. When we empathize with someone, we imagine what it is like to be in the situation of the other. Empathy helps us to align with the other person as someone worthy of our attention and care. But this exercise of imagination won't enable you to fully align with your patient's experience. The choice the patient makes can still be unfathomable to you.

You can see patients make choices that are not strategically recommended because they could have better outcomes if they were to choose differently. Moreover, you have made a professional promise to devote yourself to protect the patient from needless harm. However, to force a competent patient into making a given choice is to cause harm on an administrative level to the patient's autonomy. Recognize that supporting a right to choose is not an act of harm.

BOUNDARIES

Lakshmi and Ethan are occupational therapists working at a Cardiac Rehab facility associated with a local hospital. Ethan has been working at the facility for five years; Lakshmi has been there—her first job in health care—for five weeks. Sharing coffee during a break, Lakshmi asks Ethan for advice. She explains that, two weeks ago, she had a chance meeting with one of her patients at a local warehouse club. They chatted for a bit and went their separate ways. While it was a pleasant encounter, she says, the patient has since commented on the contents of Lakshmi's shopping cart and has been asking more and more questions about her life and family. "Of course, I'm always nice when I work with him," she says to Ethan, "but it seems like he wants to act as if we're friends. I feel that he's being intrusive. Am I wrong for feeling this way? What do I do about it?"

The right to privacy is not only possessed by patients. Health-care workers possess it as well. You will have patients who want to connect with you personally. There is a basic need for such connection, a basic need to have someone listen to you and affirm that you and your experiences matter. This is at the heart of the reason why the interpersonal level of ethical assessment is so important in care. Simply put, people need it. However, at the same time, interpersonal care does not mean that you must make yourself available to everyone who wishes to be friends or make of your life an open book.

The three levels of ethical assessment can be thought of using the imagery of distance. The administrative level is the most remote, setting abstract principles and rules that can apply to a host of particular circumstances. The strategic level is much nearer to a person who needs care but is still sufficiently hands-off to allow for a technical and rigorous analysis of the situation and of possible solutions. The interpersonal is the level of immediate proximity. This is the point of care. It is intimate. Here, at the bed side, you encounter the patient in all the patient's suffering. Moreover, you are here with the entire person, with the history and narrative that are more than this illness, more than this suffering. Some patients yearn for someone in their health-care team to recognize this aspect of them, and they want to share. Some patients want to share that side of interpersonal connection in which they bear witness to someone else. Someone like you.

Everything we do entails some risk. Moral agency means facing choices, and facing choices opens the chance to make mistakes. At the administrative level, we can make the mistakes of categorizing people unfairly, of stigmatizing people, or of affirming or denying rights and duties that should not be affirmed or denied. At the strategic level, we face the mistakes of bringing about outcomes that are undesirable and harmful, or of failing to see outcomes that could have brought about better outcomes.

At the interpersonal level, we face people in their vulnerability and connect with them there. Doing so, we open ourselves, at least empathetically, to vulnerability of our own. Mistakes of a deeply personal nature are possible here. In this chapter, we addressed the patient's need to trust, to have advocates who practice fidelity and veracity, and who protect the patient's information and dignity by respecting privacy and confidentiality. We see now that all of this amounts to being with the patient in that space of vulnerability to offer care and also to offer protection. You tend to the patient's information to maintain confidentiality and privacy. You demonstrate the qualities of trustworthiness so that the patient may feel safe in your care. You cannot hide the patient's vulnerability, but you can do your best to let the patient know that you will not use this vulnerability to hurt or gain advantage over her or him. But who protects you as you become somewhat vulnerable when you enter into this proximity of interpersonal care?

Although your professional life and social life seem to be separate, both involve *you*. Much of your social life is publicly available. Integrity is wholeness of the person. Professional integrity doesn't just apply to when you are at work. Be mindful of what you share. Your compassionate role is to be attentive to your patient. The role of listener does not mean that you are expected to offer your private life to others in your professional capacity.

TAKEAWAY

Advocacy speaks. It is a voice raised in concert with that of a patient who needs aid. As a patient exercises autonomy, an advocate proclaims this as a right. As a patient suffers, an advocate helps call for beneficent action. An advocate speaks out in nonmaleficence to prevent needless harm to the patient. For the patient who has little voice, the advocate stands for justice and lends volume to the call for aid. The advocate acts with compassionate devotion, sharing the patient's interest in being heard and aligning with the person who suffers.

Advocacy speaks. How we speak defines our advocacy. The opening phrase in health care is *first do no harm*. In the next chapter, we will explore advocacy in establishing a culture of safety.

CASE STUDIES

CASE STUDY 5.1—STRICT NPO

Lisette is a night shift nurse. One of the patients on her floor is a 38-year-old male named Ludvik. Ludvik is given the order "Strict NPO after midnight" for tests in the morning. Lisette explains the order to Ludvik as she comes on shift at 11:00 pm. She explains the NPO order to him at that time. At 1:00 am Ludvik puts on his call light and asks Lisette for ice chips. Lisette considers that a few ice chips might not have a negative impact. And yet the orders are Strict NPO, which means *nothing* orally. There is a conflict between the patient's request and the physician's orders.

What does it mean for Lisette to act as an advocate in this case? Who must she advocate for in this situation? Carefully apply the Ethical Assessment Model in order to explore this case study. Discuss (or role play) this scenario from the perspectives of the nurse and the patient.

CASE STUDY 5.2—THE PRIVATE COMPLAINT

Darleen is a 42-year-old woman. She has been seriously hurt in a motor vehicle accident. She has been stabilized in the Emergency Department and has been transferred to the ICU Trauma floor. Darleen has sustained spinal injuries. She is experiencing paralysis from the waist down. The attending neurologist is uncertain as to whether Darleen will regain the use of her legs.

Mariette is a nurse assigned to Darleen. Mariette goes into Darleen to administer medications. Darleen tells Mariette that she doesn't want to live like this. She asks if it is too late to declare herself a DNR/DNI. Mariette explains that this is possible, but the doctor has to write the order. She asks if Darleen wants her to approach the doctor. Darleen says "Yes." She adds, "And please don't tell my husband. He won't understand."

Mariette informs the doctor that Darlene has asked for a DNR/DNI order. Mariette also explains that the patient would prefer that her husband not know of this.

The next day, Darleen's husband, Beck, is in her room as Mariette comes in on a shift change. Mariette notices that Darleen looks like she's been crying. This is not unusual for this floor. But before Mariette can say anything, Beck points at the new wristband that Darleen is wearing—the one that says "DNR/DNI." He says, "What is this? Who did this to her?"

Apply the Ethical Assessment Model to this case. What should Mariette do? What does it mean for her to advocate for Darleen and respect her privacy?

CASE STUDY 5.3—IT'S STILL A 9

Charlotte is a 27-year-old female, admitted from the Emergency Department to the orthopedic floor. She has a compound fracture of the left fibula that will require surgery, which has been scheduled for tomorrow morning. While Charlotte clearly needs the surgery, she also has a history of street drug use. Her attending physician, Dr. Hunt, suspects that Charlotte will be drug seeking while she is in the hospital. He fills out the protocol for orthopedic pain management and orders the minimum pain medication.

Ying is assigned to Charlotte as her nurse for the overnight shift. Ying gives Charlotte's pain medication as prescribed. However, Charlotte is clearly uncomfortable. She rates her pain at an 8 or 9 on a 1-to-10 pain scale. Her heart rate is elevated, her blood pressure is increased. She grimaces when she attempts to reposition her leg for greater comfort. Ying calls down for increased medications to at least lower Charlotte's pain to a 5—a level at which Charlotte believes would enable her to sleep. Ying calls Dr. Hunt, but Dr. Hunt refuses to increase the dosage. As the night goes on, Charlotte's pain remains at an 8 or 9. Ying believes that Charlotte's pain is genuine.

What must Ying do in order to advocate for Charlotte? What options are available to her? Use the Ethical Assessment Model to help explore Ying's options.

REFERENCES

ARRT (2017). *ARRT standards of ethics.* St. Paul, MN: The American Registry of Radiologic Technicians. Retrieved from https://www.arrt.org/docs/default-source/Governing-Documents/arrt-standards-of-ethics.pdf?sfvrsn=12

ASHA (2016). *Code of ethics—Effective March 1, 2016.* Rockville, MD: American Speech-Language Hearing Association. Retrieved from https://www.asha.org/code-of-ethics/#sec1.2

Beauchamp, T. L., & Childress, J. F. (2013). *Principles of biomedical ethics* (7th ed.). New York, NY: Oxford University Press.

Brenan, M. (2017). Nurses keep healthy lead as most honest, ethical profession. *Gallup News.* Retrieved from http://news.gallup.com/poll/224639/nurses-keep-healthy-lead-honest-ethical-profession.aspx

Canguilhem, G. (2012). Health: Popular concept and philosophical question. In *Writings on medicine* (S. Geroulanos & T. Meyers, Trans., pp. 43–52). New York: Fordham University Press.

Eraker, S. A., Kirscht, J. P., & Becker, M. H. (1984). Understanding and improving patient compliance. *Annals of Internal Medicine, 100*(2), 258–268.

Frank, A. (2013). *The wounded storyteller: Body, illness, and ethics* (2nd ed.). Chicago: University of Chicago Press.

Kaplan, S. H., Greenfield, S., Gandek, B., Rogers, W. H., & Ware, J. E., Jr. (1996). Characteristics of physicians with participatory decision-making styles. *Annals of Internal Medicine, 124*(5), 497–504.

Mayer, R. C., Davis, J. H., & Schoorman, F. D. (1995). An integrative model of organizational trust. *Academy of Management Review, 20*(3), 709–734.

Peter, E., & Morgan, K. P. (2001). Explorations of a trust approach for nursing ethics. *Nursing Inquiry, 8*(1), 3–10.

Rutherford, M. M. (2014). The value of trust to nursing. *Nursing Economics, 32*(6), 283.

Stewart, M. A. (1995). Effective physician-patient communication and health outcomes: a review. *CMAJ: Canadian Medical Association Journal, 152*(9), 1423.

CHAPTER 6

CULTURE OF SAFETY

OBJECTIVES

After completing this chapter, you will be able to . . .

1. Define the culture of safety and recognize its prudent attributes.
2. Explain the significance of nonmaleficence in the culture of safety.
3. Demonstrate the nature of just culture and its role in the culture of safety.
4. Quantify the importance of communication and transparency in the culture of safety.
5. Discern the ways in which ignorance impacts moral responsibility.
6. Critique the roles of guilt and blame in cultivating moral agency and responsibility.
7. Contemplate the significance and possibility of forgiveness.
8. Apply the Ethical Assessment Model to chapter exercises and to real-life scenarios.

KEY TERMS

- Blame
- Culture
- Culture of safety
- Forgiveness

- Guilt
- Just culture
- Transparency

> ### *Principle 2*
>
> *Occupational therapy personnel shall refrain from actions that cause harm* (AOTA, 2015).

INTRODUCTION

Health is a process. It is not guaranteed for any of us. We are all at risk. Safety, then, is an inherent concern within health care. The adage *first, do no harm* applies to the spirit of keeping people safe. Patients are in various degrees of vulnerability. Health-care professionals face risk from different sources: accidental needle sticks, radiology, medical waste, and violent patients. The public is at some risk from communicable disease and other broad health concerns.

Safety is a highly regulated part of the healthcare industry. The interest in safeguarding people from inadvertent harm is reflected in the variety of regulatory bodies, policies, and procedures oriented around safety. These administrative- and strategic-level efforts set boundaries around safety-related issues, requiring certain behaviors when safety is at risk and prohibiting certain behaviors that would place people at risk.

The culture of safety contributes to practices that reduce errors. The principal concern is for behaviors that present risk of harm. There is a moral accountability when we deviate from practices intended to promote safety. This is why focus is drawn to cultivating a culture of safety.

Regulations, policies, and procedures facilitate safety as a matter of **culture** in part by making error reductions uniform. Beyond regulation and policy and procedure, healthcare organizations often speak of a **culture of safety**. The term speaks to an awareness that rules and regulations are only as good as people's willingness to follow them. It is one thing to have procedures in place to protect people from harm when an error occurs, but it's better to have a mindset in place that will help keep errors from happening in the first place (Scheirton, Mu, Lohman, & Cochran, 2007).

Culture of safety—to be culture—has to be a mindset. If safety is to be part of an organization's culture, then it has to be evident throughout the organization. Safety must be valued and promoted among all staff. It should also be consistently evident in policy and procedure. Safety needs to be promoted and endorsed. It needs to be known that the investment in safety is to protect everyone and that everyone shares responsibility for the culture.

Culture applies to the individual and to the collective. Ideally, accountability for safe practice should be embraced by each individual. In this ideal, a culture of safety would be a condition in which everyone possesses the mindset of protecting safety. Should an error occur, because errors will occur, the character of these virtuous people would be to learn from the error and prevent similar ones from happening

Culture refers to external (language, observances, laws) and internal (values, beliefs, attitudes) elements that are shared by people within a group and, taken together, help give a sense of the identity of people in that group as they belong with each other.

A **culture of safety** is an institutional commitment to promote the reduction of risks for harmful events.

in the future. In such an ideal culture of safety, there is little need for punitive procedures, review boards, or remediation processes. Ask these people, *How do you promote this culture?* and they will respond, *We don't. This is just who we are.*

As some procedures prove to reliably bring about better outcomes, uniformity emerges as best practice. Uniformity in practice identifies responsibilities among each individual in a healthcare team, making of each person a sentinel for patient safety. As such, a continuum of safety is established by the collective members of the healthcare team as a whole.

As an ideal, a culture of safety might be worth imagining as an aspiration. But this is not where we find ourselves. This is the task: The culture of safety demands much of us. How do we get from where we are to closer to the ideal?

NONMALEFICENCE AND OUR ERROR-PRONE WAYS

The concern for safety falls under the principle nonmaleficence. It is the commitment to protect people from inadvertent harm. Under nonmaleficence, you are accountable to be aware of safety. Nonmaleficence is the framework of the culture of safety.

By articulating the principle of nonmaleficence, we admit to our capacity to make mistakes. The principle calls upon us to avoid causing needless harm. Most of the time, we do not need to be reminded not to harm others. In Chapter 1, it was noted that we are naturally drawn to events in which harm occurs—particularly when we perceive that the harm has been intentionally caused. We are naturally harm averse to an important degree. Merely identifying nonmaleficence and beneficence as core ethical principles points to an awareness in us—one might suggest that this is common sense—that it is bad to cause needless harm.

EXERCISE

Entertain the claim that there is a human right to safety. Such a right does not mean that people have a right to expect that they are never exposed to risk. The right can indicate that people are entitled to expect that they are not unnecessarily exposed to risks of harm. How could we know if there is a right to safety? What would this right mean administratively and strategically?

We express nonmaleficence as a principle in order to set an important boundary. We are not so adept at *not* harming others that we can happily assume that we don't even need to mention it. We mention it because, even though we know in some fashion that we should not cause needless harm, we also know that needless, and often inadvertent, harm still happens.

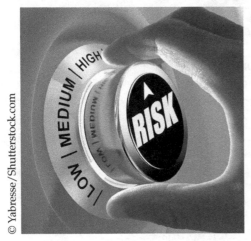

© Yabresse/Shutterstock.com

Figure 6.1

The principle of nonmaleficence is the ground of the culture of safety. It is not, however, sufficient to say that embracing this principle is enough to instill a mindset that adequately values safety. This is because the principle sets boundaries against causing harm where none exists. This is an important part of safety, but it is not the whole of it. To build toward a culture of safety, we also need to address risk of harm.

This is a subtle point. Think back to Kantian ethics. We can use the categorical imperative to demonstrate the principle of nonmaleficence. But what if we test this maxim: *If I can act in such a way as to put someone's health at risk, I will not do so in order to keep everyone safe.* While this maxim might sound noble, it seems entirely impractical. Following this maxim, we could not drive cars or prescribe medicines out of concern for slight risks of accidents or adverse side effects. In the example of giving medicines, we see that actions intended to do good sometimes present some risk of harm. Administratively, we can draw a boundary around causing harm, but we cannot draw a similar boundary around beneficent actions that present some risk of harm.

Exploring the culture of safety, then, is administratively grounded in nonmaleficence but must also entertain strategic and interpersonal considerations that pertain to managing or minimizing risks. *First do no harm* is the starting point, but healthcare must seek to help people. There are risks to what we can do to help patients. Ideally, we wish to eliminate the threat of risk wherever possible. In no way do we wish to cause harm, but risks are present; they are part of the landscape. How we navigate this landscape such that as little harm as possible is realized is an essential part of the culture of safety.

If this investment in safety is to be part of culture, then it is being promoted as a virtue. Walking through an environment in which risk is present requires habits or character traits of persistent watchfulness. Safety practices are part of your routine decision-making, your mode of operation. This becomes part of your habit. Habit is emphasized because it suggests reliability. One who has a habit of practicing safety should be less prone to error than one who does not have such a habit.

> **EXERCISE**
>
> Think about other arenas of your life: school, home, your social life. Does the culture of safety apply here as well? If not, how different would these areas be if they operated according to the culture of safety model?

JUST CULTURE

In addition to developing habits consistent with a culture of safety, it is necessary to move away from certain other habits. Of particular concern are habits in which we react to wrongdoing by passing blame or calling for punishment. In a culture of safety, identifying and preventing future errors is preferred to punishment. Stepping away from habits of seeking to pass blame is referred to as **just culture**.

There is no blame in just culture. The question to ask is *How can we fix this so that it doesn't happen again?* The aim is to continue care. The healthcare environment cannot be perfect. We can hold expectations that we strive for excellence. Virtue is excellence. You cannot have a perfect environment, but you can strive to be excellent in the environment you are in. Acting with excellence can help to improve that environment.

When we witness some errors, we might see visible harm. Seeing this can elicit an empathetic response and a moral reaction. With a moral reaction, the perception of harm is accompanied by categorization and motivation. We can categorize the harm as being someone's fault and we can be motivated to **blame**—and possibly punish—the one who is perceived as being at fault (Malle, Guglielmo, & Monroe, 2012).

One of the important steps in developing a culture of safety is steering people away from quick, empathetic reactions that can incite people to pass blame. People can fixate on blame. We're quick to judge and to defend ourselves against the possibility of being judged. Blame has a normative content—it is the passing of judgment against behaviors that have are deemed to have negative value, and against those who perform those behaviors. Judgment becomes a source of power. Blame is a judgment against the person. It is not merely a judgment against the person's act.

Just culture is a conceptual model that favors learning lessons rather than punishing people for making errors.

Blame is an assessment of a moral agent's choice or action, in which fault has been found with that agent's choice or action.

A culture of safety is incompatible with a culture of blame. In a culture of blame, people feel that they will be judged negatively, and so they will seek to protect their reputations. In a culture of safety, we want people to admit to errors and near errors (close calls or near misses). If people worry about being blamed, they will be less likely to report errors, fearing that they will be adversely judged. Further, if people fear blame and punishment, they might seek to protect themselves by doing less. Patient outcomes could suffer as professionals withhold their own actions that might present some risk.

A culture of blame can also prove to be divisive. In efforts to escape blame, people can try to pass blame off on each other or isolate those they blame or those who have blamed them. People can try to use blame as a way to advance their own personal agendas.

We don't want to be blamed, but we want to be acknowledged for what we do well. To seek acknowledgment but not blame is to value only half the truth, however. If we are to acknowledge good acts, then we must also take note of errors. There is value in recognizing both, but this recognition is hampered if we fear blame.

EXERCISE

Leo is a nurse, working a medical floor. He has orders to administer 12.5 mg of promethazine for Loretta, a 51-year-old female who is complaining of nausea. The order is for 12.5 mg, the vial contains 25 mg. Leo draws up the medication. As he administers the promethazine into the IV, he and Loretta talk about her children. After he administers the drug he realizes that, instead of drawing up 12.5 mg and then wasting 12.5 mg, he administered all 25 mg. Loretta is comfortable, though a little lightheaded. Discuss what Leo should do, promoting a culture of safety. Leo made a mistake. Did he act unethically? Use the Ethical Assessment Model to explore Leo's mistake and the options available to him.

COMMUNICATION IN THE CULTURE OF SAFETY

The culture of safety relies on communication. If individuals do not effectively communicate with each other, then patients or coworkers might be put at risk. Errors and near errors need to be communicated. People need to feel that they can come forward with concerns, questions, and reports of mistakes without fear. What we learn from mistakes can be taught to other people. Any mistake that one person can make can be made by another person in similar circumstances. Communicating errors contributes to safety, at the very least, by building awareness (da Costa et al., 2017).

The culture of safety will include care in identifying patients, double-checking orders, and other means of effective communication. These measures help to protect patients and improve outcomes. Practicing the *Rights of Medication Administration*, for example, avoids medication errors (CDC, n.d.).

Reduction in errors and minimizing risks and the harm that would come from them are the two main goals in a culture of safety. There are a variety of ways to strategically target these goals. The SBAR structure is an example of an effort to standardize communication. As communication improves, errors that would come from miscommunication are reduced and minimize risks that would come from such errors.

It is vital that people take responsibility for what they do. A just culture values honest discovery and disclosure of facts. Revealing the truth about errors and near errors is more important than passing blame. The truth is essential to the discovery of ways to improve procedures, education, and policies. Disseminating information pertinent to risk and safety does more to improve health outcomes than does blaming people for their errors.

So, what happens when there is an error? *Just culture* discerns between human error and risks. Investigations are undertaken to make sure that due diligence has been followed in adhering to a culture of safety.

Not everything needs to be sirens and lights and a police escort. You can promote a culture of safety by adhering to guidelines and anticipating the potential for risks. Everything is done to minimize errors as much as possible. There are accepted practices that, if followed, are intended to eliminate chances for errors to occur. Safety procedures are designed to direct attention to possible risks and plans to manage them. When errors occur, we can investigate to determine the source of the error. Where was the breakdown? Was the error avoidable? The point of investigation is not to assign blame, but to identify what can be done to ensure better outcomes.

The commitment to safety demonstrates value. The commitment extends from recognizing a duty to keep patients, health-care professionals, and the public safe. Because of this duty, the healthcare industry is very regulated with respect to safety precautions.

The lifeblood of culture is communication. The ideas, beliefs, and values of culture all need to be spread in order to be shared. All of the external elements are media of communication through which messages about value and belonging are disseminated. In a culture of safety, where minimization of risk is a central value, effective communication is important as a means to avoid harm for coworkers as well as for patients.

ERROR AND IGNORANCE

We saw in Chapter 3 that Kant described three degrees of moral failure. He described these three—frailty, impurity, and wickedness—as aspects of our "propensity to evil" (Kant, 1960). If you find that Kant sounds harsh here, you're to be excused. "Evil" seems a strong word to apply at this point. We do not offer the principle of nonmaleficence because we are convinced that people are evil and look to harm others at every opportunity. The evidence is that we have a natural inclination to avoid harm. And yet, we still cause harm to others and to ourselves. There are many reasons why harm happens. Kant might well be able to explain some of these. We will turn our attention in this chapter to other reasons for the harm we cause—error and ignorance.

Errors happen. Mistakes will be made. Articulating nonmaleficence as a principle is a way of setting a reminder: *You have the ability to harm as well as to benefit. You can be dangerous. Take care in what you do.*

There's a difference between what you should have known and what you couldn't have known. Both can be described as ignorance, but blame accrues to these differently. Suppose an adverse event happens and harm occurs. For instance, imagine that a patient is treated with penicillin and has an anaphylactic reaction. Had it been known that the patient was allergic to penicillin, it certainly would not have been prescribed. Consider now two variations on this scenario. In one variation, no one, not even the patient, knew that there was an allergy to penicillin. In the other variation, imagine that information about an allergy to penicillin is available but no one accessed that information. In the first variation, the allergy could not have been known. In the second, it should have been known.

EXERCISE

Imagine the scenario in the example just given in which an allergy to penicillin is on a patient's record, but no one accesses the information. In a culture of safety that practices just culture, how should this error be addressed. Use the Ethical Assessment Model to explore options.

There is something distressing about confronting your own ignorance. There can be some comfort in recognizing that a point of ignorance could not have been avoided—you couldn't have known. Still, you can be hard on yourself. You care; you wish you could have done better. Maybe you did all you could, but if only you had known . . . . Then consider the condition in which you realize that you should have known better. This can be humiliating. You should have known. It will feel punitive if you feel that you could have avoided an error if only you caught a detail that you missed.

ETHICAL MISTAKES

In healthcare, it is important to protect the privacy of patients. Information is held in confidence. Care is given with sensitivity to privacy. Much of the way we interact with patients is held in areas that are not made open to the public. At the same time, the work we do needs to be effectively and appropriately communicated.

Accidents happen. Mistakes are made. Ethically, we can see a difference between the two. Accidents happen despite our best efforts to prevent harm. You know that accidents will occur, but you cannot know when or how they occur. A mistake, on the other hand, is avoidable. When there is a mistake, there is a situation in which someone should have known better.

The Ethical Assessment Model provides a tool to identify the ways in which we can assess mistakes. We can fall short of gathering situational and background information and make mistakes because there was information that we could have known but missed. We can miss important insight from assessing the administrative, strategic, or interpersonal levels. This model is not a guide toward perfect action. It is a guideline that can help to enhance your ability to assess, and act in, a moral situation.

EXERCISE

You can do your best to assess a moral situation and still be somewhat unsatisfied with the outcomes or with your action. Even though you did your best, you feel you could have done better. This does not necessarily mean that you were wrong. What is the difference between an ethical mistake and feeling that you could have done better?

GUILT AND REMORSE

Guilt is a feeling of remorse for an act that one believes has violated a moral standard and that one is responsible for that act.

We all make mistakes. Even in a culture of safety, errors will still occur. Even in a just culture, there will be blame. It may be self-imposed blame, and it may be all the worse for being self-imposed.

Guilt has two manifestations. The first is what we experience when we recognize that we have made a mistake and feel some wrongdoing for it. There is an emotional response in which one acknowledges blame for the wrong that has occurred. Guilt, in this way, is a form of suffering. Second, guilt can have a normative aspect that warns against repeating a mistake in the future. The emotional suffering of guilt, or the cognitive awareness of the mistake, can serve as a lesson: You don't want to have this experience again.

Guilt can be felt when mistakes haven't been made. This happens when we feel that we have not met expectations. Guilt, then, can be a response to perceived failure. We can perceive guilt because of being part of an event that did not turn out optimally.

Feeling guilty does not necessarily mean that you deserve to feel guilty. As self-suffering, guilt is what you feel. Guilt arises with the recognition that events have not happened as you would have them happen. It associates with a disappointment in events that have to you some kind of moral worth. Because there is failure in this part of your moral experience, the perception of guilt arises. You might not be the cause of this failure, but you can feel guilty even so. Seeing this, we realize that guilt is not necessarily a judgment about what you deserve.

As moral agents, we seek a sense of significance in our lives. The feeling of guilt shows us that, to some extent, we can do better. This feeling has normative value because it can cause you to step back and evaluate your circumstances and your behavior. This can inspire critical thinking and ethical assessment. This is the irony of guilt: for all that it feels like a negative moral evaluation, it can have a positive ethical effect.

The culture of safety aims to prevent errors. As guilt manifests when our expectations for good outcomes don't emerge, the culture of safety helps to reduce circumstances in which guilt—itself a form of suffering—occurs.

After examining just culture, one might wonder what happens to responsibility and accountability once we call for an environment without blame. To answer this, we explore the nature of moral responsibility.

MORAL AGENCY AND RESPONSIBILITY

A moral agent is one who bears responsibility. Responsibility extends from your awareness that there is something morally significant at stake and that you have choices that bear on these stakes. Part of your awareness extends to recognizing that your choice and the action that follows from it matter as well. Saying that your choice and action matter—that you bear responsibility—means that assessment of your choices and actions are possible. So, we can say that your action was permissible or impermissible, right or wrong, acceptable or unacceptable. You acted well or you should have done better. At the outset, it would seem that two types of reaction are possible when your choices and actions are assessed. We can *praise* a moral agent who does well. We can offer *blame* when a moral agent should have done better.

One of the earliest known discussions of praise and blame is found in Aristotle's *Nicomachean Ethics*. In this exploration, Aristotle draws attention to the importance of personal control in choosing. Personal control means making your choice willingly and being aware of the ramifications of the choice (Aristotle, 2002). Personal control amounts to determining the degree to which an error is avoidable or unavoidable.

There are factors that mitigate responsibility by eroding your personal control. Ignorance means that you are unaware of all the options available to you, or you are unaware of the ramifications of following through on the choice you are considering. When ignorance is unavoidable—when you couldn't have known—responsibility is diffused.

EXERCISE

Can you identify any other factors that might erode personal control and mean that you bear less responsibility for a mistake or wrong act?

If you concentrate on seeing things the way they are instead of being distracted by what you want to see, you will be less inclined to focus on where blame should be placed. Part of the reason you want to lay blame is because your own expectations were disappointed. When people disappoint you—i.e., let you down—you might feel inclined to hold them at fault for your own disappointment. Letting go of the expectations doesn't mean letting go of standards; it means taking on a view to see circumstances for what they are. From this vantage point, you are better able to see what needs to be done in this situation as well as identify errors that might have occurred. Taking this view moves you away from a framework in which you seek to associate blame for the actions of others. It becomes more focused on having a practical impact. Just culture encourages an attitude in which the focus is placed on fixing errors and preventing their recurrence. The focus is not on punishment, but on correction.

In the culture of safety, you have to acknowledge your errors or near errors. This is a form of transparency. You are a participant in the culture of safety. This culture is for everyone. Where errors occur, the impact can be felt elsewhere. Raising attention to this error of yours can forestall harm to someone else. Raising attention to your error can also help others learn from your mistake, improving safety throughout the culture.

As observed earlier, we often adopt a defensive attitude toward blame. Consequences can stem from blame. If you recognize that you are blameworthy for your action, you might feel a mix of reactions. You might feel guilty. You might feel for the well-being of anyone who might suffer the consequences of your error. You might recognize that you have to own this error.

Think of communicating errors as a test of character. It is comparatively easy to do the right thing when circumstances are good and there is little pressure. But what do you do when circumstances are bad, you're feeling pressure, and you've made a mistake?

EXERCISE

Reflect on a mistake that you have made and for which you feel some guilt. Imagine that someone else had made this same mistake. Would you blame this person in the same way that you hold yourself guilty? Do you suppose you are more inclined to be harder on yourself or on someone else?

Having made a mistake, you face the prospect of blame. Even in a just culture, blame can still arise as you blame yourself for your own error. Blame hurts, regardless of the source. It brings you low. It can make you feel discredited. It can make you wonder about your suitability for your role. You might feel that you will be singled out and isolated for your error. By internalizing the blame—by feeling discreditable—you isolate yourself.

In the case of a medical error, it's the patient who will suffer the consequences. Your intention is to do good for your patient, to be beneficent. But mistakes happen. Harm—or the risk of harm—arises.

Maybe you'd like to go back in time to take away the mistake. You dig through *Could I have known better?* and *Should I have known better?* You feel that you have to revisit the bad in this way. The first response to the perception of error is to examine your own agency. Was this mistake avoidable?

When outcomes do not match your intentions, the first step in moral agency should be to resort to this line of inquiry as an algorithm. First ask, *Could I have known?* If the answer is *Yes*, then ask *Should I have known?* This is simple but isn't easy. By asking these questions, you expose yourself to guilt and blame. But, by asking these questions, you put yourself in position to identify your own role in the error and, by extension, examine your moral agency. You learn something about your integrity in the moment this error occurred and in the moment that you reflect on, and learn from, this error. How you answer the questions in this model helps to locate yourself in this situation. Proper use of this model requires veracity. Be honest with yourself as you ask these questions. Though blame might be at risk, the purpose of the model is to explain, not to blame.

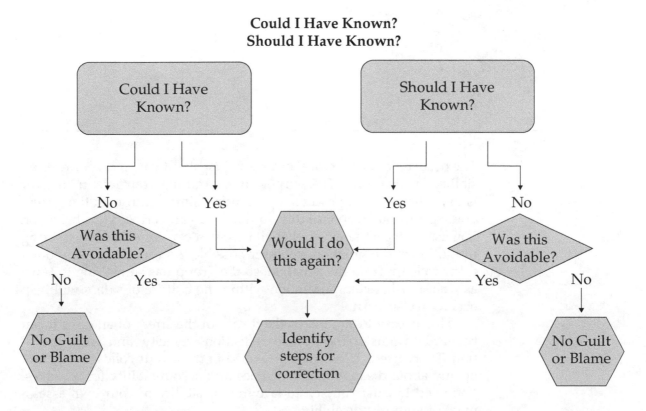

Could I Have Known?
Should I Have Known?

Figure 6.2 Could/Should Model

Using this model, if your answer to both questions is *Yes,* then ask yourself a third question: *Would I do this again?* At this instance, this algorithm can be a tool for self-correction. One of our motivations to learn is to realize that we have room for improvement. You can't grow until you've made mistakes. How do you move forward from here?

If you can honestly say *No* to the first question, then you realize that you are not at fault. The error should not be taken as a judgment against your moral agency. You might not bear moral responsibility for this error, but you remain a moral agent now. Who is feeling responsible for this error? What does this person need from you? Can you be a sounding board, a source of comfort, a reminder for better action in the future?

EXERCISE

What does it mean to know? Imagine a scenario in which you can see a possibility that someone might act in error. You see this potential and could speak up to prevent the error, but you believe that this person knows better. You say nothing. You are horrified, then, to see that the other person did, in fact, commit the error you thought wasn't going to occur. Could you have known? Should you have known? Discuss.

The occurrence of a medical error isn't just about you and your responsibility for that error. The purpose of examining your role in an error is to participate in a process of preventing similar errors in the future. You assess your responsibility so that you can correct your behavior. You assess the situation so that all involved can communicate to bring resolution to the situation wherever possible. As you might have something to learn from the situation, so the group has something to learn as well. Further communication within the culture of safety will help everyone else learn.

This is easy to say, but in the throes of the stress of an error it can be hard to muster the needed reflection, veracity, and communication. There needs to be trust. You need to trust your colleagues to talk openly about disappointed outcomes and accountability for mistakes. You need to trust yourself to face the possibility of your own assessment of your responsibility.

It is possible to look at guilt as part of a process of negative conditioning. In this view, guilt is a form of suffering that creates a disincentive against certain actions. If you made a mistake and feel guilty for that mistake, the attending suffering of that feeling of guilt can make you vigilant about not making this kind of mistake again.

Guilt can be used to enhance ethical competency. There is something useful in the capacity to acknowledge error and commit to correct it. Guilt itself isn't to be valued, but what you do with it can bring value. Where an error has occurred, guilt can inspire us ethically to investigate and productively address the situation. In this way, guilt can lead to actions that are worthy of praise.

EXERCISE

See how the model just presented can be used in conjunction with the Ethical Assessment Model in cases where a mistake has occurred.

Guilt, as a moral reaction, is highly individualized. An action that might make one person feel guilty might not make someone else feel similarly guilty. The action might be the same, but the personal response might vary. Guilt, like empathy, helps to set a pathway to travel through your own, personal moral world. Empathy draws you toward those whose suffering compels you. Guilt steers you away from repeating actions that you associate with moral fault. This individualized pathway is your inclination to move morally. As this might be your perspective, this is a form of bias. Ethically, you can do better. This is not necessarily to say that your perspective is wrong, but that there is more to see and you might find better ways to act if you critically explore your own reactions in light of other views. It is important to recognize that your feeling of guilt—powerful though it may be—is not the only way to view a moral issue.

Guilt is a feeling that you have responsibility for an undesired outcome. It is the crossfire between your intention and the outcome. While we have so far associated this feeling with a mistake like a medical error, it's important to notice that feelings can sometimes arise from a different kind of mistake—mistakes in perception. When there are undesired outcomes that elicit our empathy, we are motivated to assign responsibility. We are prone to assign this responsibility to ourselves even if we really have no causal role in the outcome. The mere association with a situation in which harm results can motivate us to feel guilt. In other words, we can feel guilt even if we didn't actively do anything to contribute to the outcome. Here again, is the need for ethical analysis. The mere feeling of guilt might not be an indication of wrongdoing.

At its best, guilt serves constructive criticism. At its worst, guilt can be a source of self-punishment in which you only see judgment against yourself. Should you feel this way, remind yourself gently that ethics is not a matter of branding people for their behavior. Ethics is an essential part of a process of personal and social growth. Where guilt has a role in ethics is at its best use. Take the constructive criticism and allow it to become a means to gain perspective and to improve.

EXERCISE

Consider how often people assign blame to others and offer it as constructive criticism. How often do people assign blame destructively instead? What is the appeal to using guilt and blame to discredit, isolate, or categorize people?

We don't pay much attention to what we do well. When things are going well, we regard our circumstances as normal or 'as they ought to be'. When harm or threat of harm arises, we take notice. Threats of disruption to what we take for granted grabs our attention. We are more attentive to wrong than we are to right. And so, many of us tend to be quicker to offer blame than to offer praise (Malle, Guglielmo, & Monroe, 2012).

Moral judgments are not always negative. We can acknowledge good behavior and take satisfaction in it, just as we can feel guilt or pass blame for bad behavior. There is nuance to our moral assessments. Acknowledgment is not the exact opposite of blame.

Acknowledgment, like guilt, can be a tool for growth. Where guilt can be a tool for correction, acknowledgment serves to encourage continued enhancement of one's ethical competency.

An assessment involves acknowledgment of what happened and what was possible. Assessment is evidence-gathering. In assessing one's actions in a moral event, we gather evidence and review what worked and what didn't and what met standards and what didn't. We also review for evidence of personal control. The act of gathering evidence can be value-neutral. There is no judgment, just an effort to build awareness of what happened and what could have happened. Where the assessment assigns no blame or praise, and yet there are lessons learned from the evidence, then there is acknowledgment.

In order to acknowledge what has been done, what has been done must be made known. For the sake of a culture of safety, information has to be made available. Transparency is needed.

TRANSPARENCY

Veracity applies to all matters of truth-telling. **Transparency** is an approach to honesty. Being forthcoming, not withholding information. Not filtering information. Report back what you observe. Report what you have done. This is a special approach to veracity.

Veracity is a virtue associated with a dedication to the truth. Veracity has no room for deceit. Truth is told, and it is told without the intent to mislead or coerce. Transparency adds an expectation of full disclosure of the truth.

Transparency carries an image of clarity. Make it easy for someone to see the facts. Not seeking praise or blame, you report information that is needed for patient care and for the continuum of care.

Transparency carries a note of trustworthiness. Not only does it constitute disclosure, it also demonstrates the absence of any hidden agenda. If you are transparent, no scrutiny will turn up any undisclosed information. Transparency wards off conflict. Everything relevant has been put forward.

Transparency is an ethical skill. Being truthful. Reporting what you've seen and done. On a strategic level, it is meaningful because it affects patient outcomes.

Transparency can be useful as a way to talk through a problem. It can be used to invite participation and collaboration. If the information is there, we can confer and talk about it. Transparency has useful implications for strategic-level decision-making.

Transparency describes the disclosure of truth, providing clarity about what is known and revealing the lack of any hidden agenda.

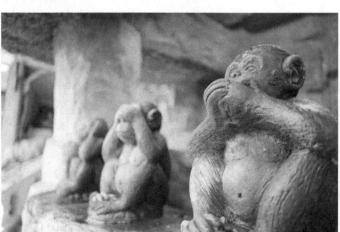

Figure 6.3 This is not transparency

© Surachet Jo/Shutterstock.com

Raising a call to establish a culture of safety amounts to a call for some degree of cultural change. Bringing about cultural change takes a multidimensional approach. Regulations and policies can set requirements to maintain a safe working environment, safe handling of hazardous substances, protection of sensitive information.

Transparency aligns with the culture of safety due to the need for full and free disclosure of information to prevent risk and promote best practices for safety. Transparency particularly aligns with just culture and helps to reinforce the call for nonpunitive structures. Promoting transparency promotes accountability: everyone is expected to be open and honest about their actions. But accountability need not be synonymous with punishment. The fear of punishment provides a disincentive to transparency.

FORGIVENESS

If the emphasis on the culture of safety is meant to be nonpunitive and we are inclined to blame and feel guilt, then the culture surrounding safety must include room for forgiveness. As we promote a just culture, we must realize that we cannot produce an ideal culture in which no one is ever inclined to blame someone else. Realizing that we are prone to judge and blame, we then recognize the value of forgiveness in the culture of safety.

Forgiveness is absence of judgment or blame toward one who has been accused of doing wrong.

Forgiveness doesn't have to mean forgetting. When one forgives, one affirms the value of the person who is being forgiven and recognizes that the value of this person is independent of any wrongdoing that this person may have performed. In short, no judgment is held against the person who is forgiven even though it may still be important to hold some judgment against this person's act. In this way, a mistake can be brought to light as inspiration to refine a safety protocol even while the person who made the mistake is not blamed.

Forgiveness can involve any of three elements: an act of wrongdoing, one who asks for forgiveness, and one who grants forgiveness. Not all three of these elements need to be in place. One might ask forgiveness for an act that hasn't been judged wrong. Someone who does wrong might not ask forgiveness. Even so, someone might still offer forgiveness for that person's act.

EXERCISE

A patient is in transport and is overcome with sudden nausea. The patient vomits while in the wheelchair. As you're cleaning up, the patient apologizes profusely. The patient was ill and wasn't in a position to make a choice not to vomit. This is not at all blameworthy. Should you forgive the patient? Use the Ethical Assessment Model to determine how should you respond.

But forgiveness always requires the act of the person who offers forgiveness. It seems plain to say that forgiveness cannot occur until it is offered by someone.

There is some question as to when forgiveness is appropriate. Must someone earn your forgiveness before you offer it? If so, what must you see in that person before forgiveness is an appropriate response? There is an alternative view in which forgiveness is seen as an act of grace. It is given, not merited.

EXERCISE

Think about when forgiveness is appropriate. Do you believe it should be earned before it is given? Do you believe that it can be given as a gesture of grace? Is it possible to take both views? Discuss.

Forgiveness serves the purpose of reconciliation. If someone has done wrong, judgments about that act might bring discredit and isolation to that person. Forgiveness removes this judgment against the person though not necessarily against the act. In salvaging the person from the act, forgiveness reaches out to the person to offer continued acceptance and belonging.

It can be hard for us to separate an act from the person who performs it. It can be hard not to judge. There is power in holding a grudge and maintaining resentment. This is the power of isolation, of holding someone at a distance. It is a measure of seeking control. But there is also power in forgiveness. Forgiveness is a choice, and here there is also control. Forgiveness holds the power to bring people together, to work together, and to act toward mutual goals.

Forgiveness also serves the one who forgives. When you hold judgment against someone else, you isolate yourself from that person. Your act of forgiveness not only reconciles that person to you, it also reconciles you to that person. Ultimately, forgiveness is an interpersonal act that brings people together.

Reconciliation doesn't mean that you have to like somebody. A relationship doesn't have to be fully restored to what it was before an act of wrongdoing occurred. With an act of wrongdoing, the relationship can change. With an act of forgiveness, the relationship changes again.

It might not return to what it was before the wrongdoing. Forgiveness doesn't mean forgetting. Reconciliation is the sense of knowing the difference between an act and a person. It is a restoration of respect for the person.

SELF-FORGIVENESS

It is possible to forgive someone who has not asked for forgiveness. One might see that someone has merited forgiveness even without asking for it. Or, alternatively, one might offer forgiveness as an act of grace. Consider what this means in the case of self-forgiveness. Self-forgiveness is only an issue when you continue to hold yourself in judgment. You are not inclined to ask for your own forgiveness, holding yourself in blame.

If you hold yourself in blame, you do not see yourself as worthy of respect. Self-judgment without forgiveness isolates. Reconciliation is a means of restoring self-respect.

The image of self-blame is one of a fragmented self. An individual split into two halves: one that judges, one that bows under the weight of judgment. Return, then, to the notion of integrity as wholeness. Your profession and the people you serve need you as a whole person. Self-forgiveness is essential to your integrity.

There is probably little controversy in saying that we should all develop the skills of practicing self-forgiveness. One hard part of the task is summoning the motivation and will to forgive. The other hard part is figuring out how to practice self-forgiveness.

Forgiveness and trust belong together. The act of forgiveness involves an act of restoring some level of trust. You might not trust the forgiven person in quite the same way, but you discover some way to find trust in this person again. The same goes for self-forgiveness (Hall & Fincham, 2005; Holmgren, 1998). Can you find a way to trust yourself again? Can you trust yourself to perform your professional tasks?

On the whole, there can be a lot of work in forgiving. Forgiveness is a choice. You can choose to wait for someone to earn your forgiveness—to prove that they are worthy of your trust again. You can choose to offer your forgiveness as grace—to take the risk of placing some trust in this person once more. Both choices entail risk. To trust means to reach out. To forgive means that you are reaching out to someone who has perhaps violated your trust already. When trust is hard there is a fear for security. When trust is hard, identify the concern. Identify the fear.

A culture of safety is a culture in which risks of harm are identified. The culture of safety operates on many levels, involving many people. As culture, it is an effort involving many people who can support each other and hold each other accountable. Still, a culture is made up of individuals. Individuals rely on each other for belonging and support. And yet, the individual possesses a unique perspective, reactions, and will. Forgiveness holds comparable value for the individual that just culture holds for the culture of safety. What lessons do each have for the other? What do we see in the challenges of forgiveness that should be accounted for in working to build a culture of safety and just culture? What do we see in the structures of a culture of safety that can help us learn to forgive others and ourselves?

TAKEAWAY

You don't just hold your license as your own private possession. You are holding it for other people. This is a trust for individual and public safety. The duties of your role, the skills of your profession are for the good of others.

The environment in which you practice these skills is one in which people are at risk. Your skills can help to address and prevent suffering. Not only do you use your clinical skills, you also use your ethical competency. See how your mindset and your attitude toward responsibility can contribute to the safety of your patients, your coworkers, and yourself.

CASE STUDIES

CASE STUDY 6.1—ALBUTEROL HISTORY

Zane is a 6-year-old male who is being admitted for a tonsillectomy. He is in the pre-op area, accompanied by his mother, Johanna. Jose is the nurse and is performing the pre-op assessment and medication reconciliation. Zane and his mother are clearly anxious, which Jose notes. Jose also notes no current medications and no known allergies, per the mother's statement.

Post-op, Zane presents minor stridor. Zane's post-op nurse, Karen, notifies the anesthesiologist who orders an albuterol nebulizer treatment. Hailey, a respiratory therapist, arrives to administer the nebulizer. As soon as Hailey puts the face mask over Zane's nose and mouth, the stridor becomes severe. Zane is in respiratory distress. Johanna is upset and demands, "What did you give him?" Hailey explains that she administered an albuterol nebulizer. "On no!" says Johanna, "The last time he had that, he reacted just like this!"

After Zane recovers from this respiratory event, Karen calls Hailey and asks about the incident. Both confirm that they have no notation that Zane had any known allergy to albuterol. Yet his mother was adamant that he'd had this reaction to albuterol before. Karen calls Jose, who recalls that there was no mention from Johanna or Zane of any allergy. He believes that he is clear in his recall.

Use the Ethical Assessment Model. Did anyone do anything wrong here? Could Karen or Hailey have known not to administer albuterol? Could Jose have conducted the interview any differently? In the interest of a culture of safety, should anything be done differently in the future?

(Continued)

CASE STUDY 6.2—THE INCESSANT CALL LIGHT

Roland and Tricia are having a discussion at the nurse's station. They are discussing their frustration with Peter, an 88-year-old male, who puts on his call light every 15 minutes. His requests range from claiming to be too cold, too hot, wanting ice chips, complaining about the arrangement of his room, and more. Peter's wife of 64 years, Irene, has been with him all day. She has apologized profusely each time Peter calls for seemingly no good reason.

Roland is at the end of his shift and at the end of his patience. He makes a disparaging joke about Peter's age and doesn't notice that the door to Peter's room has opened. As Roland finishes his joke, he turns and sees Irene, who is leaving for the day. She makes eye contact with Roland and Tricia, flushes with embarrassment, and quickly turns for the elevators.

Use the Ethical Assessment Model to assess how Peter and Tricia should have handled this situation. Use this model to assess how they should act now.

CASE STUDY 6.3—PPE

Nigel is a 56-year-old male diagnosed with tuberculosis. He is in an airborne isolation room. There is a blue sign on Nigel's door, specifying what protective personal equipment (PPE) is required for entry to the room.

Sadie is a nursing assistant. She enters Nigel's room to get a set of vitals. Sadie listens at the door and hears no sound. Believing that the patient is quiet and sleeping, she chooses not to don the PPE. She has many tasks to perform and doesn't want to be slowed down by the PPE. She thinks that, since Nigel is sleeping, she can take his vitals quickly and be on her way.

Use the Ethical Assessment Model to evaluate Sadie's choice to not wear the PPE.

REFERENCES

AOTA. (2015). *Occupational therapy code of ethics*. Bethesda, MD: AOTA.

Aristotle, & Sachs, J. (2002). *Nicomachean ethics* (pp. 1110a–1111b). Newbury, MA: Focus Pub./R. Pullinst.

CDC. (n.d.). *Vaccine administration*. Atlanta, GA: CDC. Retrieved from https://www.cdc.gov/vaccines/pubs/pinkbook/downloads/vac-admin.pdf

da Costa, T. D., Santos V. E. P., Junior, M. A. F., Vitor, A. F., de Oliveira Salvador, P. T. C., Alves, K. Y. A. (2017). Evaluation procedures in health: Perspective of nursing care in patient safety. *Applied Nursing Research, 35*, 71–76.

Hall, J. H., & Fincham, F. D. (2005). Self-forgiveness: The stepchild of forgiveness research. *Journal of Social and Clinical Psychology, 24*(5), 621–637.

Holmgren, M. R. (1998). Self-forgiveness and responsible moral agency. *The Journal of Value Inquiry, 32*(1), 75–91.

Kant, I. (1960). *Religion within the limits of reason alone* (T. M. Greene & H. H. Hudson, Trans.). New York: Harper and Brothers.

Malle, B. F., Guglielmo, S., & Monroe, A. E. (2012). Moral, cognitive, and social: The nature of blame. *Social Thinking and Interpersonal Behaviour, 313*–331.

Scheirton, L. S., Mu, K., Lohman, H., & Cochran, T. M. (2007). Error and patient safety: Ethical analysis of cases in occupational and physical therapy practice. *Medicine, Health Care and Philosophy, 10*(3), 301.

CHAPTER 7

MORAL DEJECTION

OBJECTIVES

After completing this chapter, you will be able to . . .

1. Describe empathy and explain its role in the various types of moral dejection.

2. Describe moral distress and decipher contributing factors in the workplace.

3. Identify the nature of an ethical dilemma, and scrutinize the effects of moral residue.

4. Explore the difference between compassion and empathy, and the role of compassion in mitigating moral dejection.

5. Discuss techniques for teaching compassion to students in nursing and allied health programs.

6. Apply the Ethical Assessment Model to chapter exercises and to real-life scenarios.

KEY TERMS

- Compassion fatigue
- Empathy fatigue
- Ethical dilemma
- Gratification

- Moral dejection
- Moral distress
- Moral residue

INTRODUCTION

Let's start with some perspective. In 2016, over 2.8 million registered nurses were employed in the United States (U.S. Bureau of Labor Statistics, 2018e), nearly 1.5 million certified nursing assistants (U.S. Bureau of Labor Statistics, 2018g), over 200,000 physical therapists (U.S. Bureau of Labor Statistics, 2018c), approximately 150,000 nurse practitioners (U.S. Bureau of Labor Statistics, 2018f), over 125,000 respiratory therapists (U.S. Bureau of Labor Statistics, 2018d), nearly 120,000 occupational therapists (U.S. Bureau of Labor Statistics, 2018b), and over 100,000 physician assistants (U.S. Bureau of Labor Statistics, 2018a). In the same year, there were over 35 million hospital admissions in the United States (AHA Hospital Statistics, 2018). This figure does not account for patients not admitted to the hospital, nor those seen in primary care or urgent care facilities. The point is that patient volume is huge. These numbers reinforce what we all know: Nurses and allied health professionals are busy and stressed for time on the job.

In addition to demands on time, the work itself is stressful. The suffering felt by patients can trigger empathy responses in health-care workers, which, as we have seen, is a response of mirrored suffering. Moreover, the work is focused on the suffering or the cause of suffering of those patients, adding an emotional investment in patient outcomes. In sum, ingredients for stress on the job are inherently present.

EXERCISE

Every chapter in this book opens with an excerpt from a professional code of ethics pertaining to the topic of the chapter. Investigate codes of ethics in nursing or another allied health profession on the topic of moral self-care. In the pursuit of integrity, what must you do to take care of yourself?

In this chapter, we turn to the moral cost of job stress and burnout on nurses and allied health professionals. Not only is this attention warranted because of the personal toll it takes, but the moral cost also impacts patient safety (Maiden, Georges, & Connelly, 2011).

AGENCY, GRATIFICATION, AND CONFLICT

A moral agent recognizes that there is a choice to be made, that there is some moral weight hanging on this choice, and that there is some responsibility that appends to making this choice. You act agentially when you consciously set yourself the task of assessing your circumstances and arrive at an intervention that you deem to be consistent with good, responsible action.

One feature of moral agency is narrative. We each craft accounts of ourselves in an effort to make sense of ourselves as agents within the world. We develop accounts to answer fundamental questions: *What is happening? What is my world? What's my role in all of this?* This last question arises from our awareness of ourselves as agents. In crafting an account of ourselves as moral agents, we further ask *What have I done to contribute to the circumstances I see? What should I do now?*

The next to last question especially speaks to our awareness of our moral agency. We commonly look to the world we see, expecting to see signs of our own involvement. *Things are the way they are in part because of me,* says the moral agent. Those of us with inflated senses of self see our imprint—accurately or not—on many of the good things we find in the world. Some of us—perhaps all of us at times—seek to avoid culpability for undesirable circumstances that we might have been involved in. Many of us, when confronted with circumstances we deeply do not wish to experience, find ways to blame ourselves. Again, this blame can be accurately assigned or not. These stories are crafted from some combination of the conscious, decision-making, agential aspects of our minds and from the intuitive, emotional, reactive aspects of our minds. This means that our explanations are not always thoroughly rational. Notice, for instance, that we are not always rational in our assessment of blame. Sometimes, we blame ourselves harshly for events that we could not have prevented or over-inflate our role in events that don't turn out as we had hoped.

At the same time, a compelling narrative often involves a rational effort to make sense of disparate and competing emotional responses and motivations. In this narrative effort, we can bring in the capacity of the conscious mind to modulate our emotional reactions. We can set our sights on abstract notions of moral objectives and principles.

Narrative refers to an effort to find and affirm value in who we are and in what we do. Through narrative, we seek a way of describing our lives and places in the world that makes a certain amount of sense, even though we can certainly craft explanations that stretch credibility. More, we seek ways of explaining our lives that show that we belong and that we have significance. Accounting for our moral agency speaks to our relationships with others in this world, in which we fill some role that builds connections that are useful, even necessary, to others.

The narratives we tell are more than voice overs, more than fiction. This isn't merely story-telling. We don't find value in our lives simply by deciding that we have found it. We need to develop an account of that describes the significance of our lives. This account may depend on a synchrony among our perceptions of actions, feelings, beliefs, motivations, aspirations, and from the reactions and responses from other people as well as from conditions in the world. We act in this world. We tell our narratives through our deeds as well as through our explanations. Indeed, our explanations serve to add meaning to—or interpret—the actions that we have taken. And so, we take a vested interest in seeing that our actions have some sort of moral significance. We wish to see—need to see—that the intentions behind our efforts to act morally bear fruit in the world. We want to be able to offer a narrative of helping to bring about a world that better suits our moral sensibilities.

EXERCISE

Describe what is important to you. Who are you? Who do you want to be? What do you want to contribute to the world? What stands in your way? What frustrates you? Look over your responses to these questions and think about the image you have of yourself as an agent in this world.

Moreover, we are participants in this world. Our narratives seek to grasp the manner in which we belong. This belonging is not an abstract recognition of a shared place in the world, but an awareness of participation. We have and need relationships with others. Recognizing ourselves as moral agents, part of our stories addresses how our actions and attitudes impact those with whom we are in relationship. We also look to the way that others in relationship with us serve to address—or fail to address—our needs. Again, this is more than an abstract, intellectual exercise. We invest significant emotional content in our experience of moral agency.

In Chapter 1, we identified emotional content in initial moral judgment. When you form a judgment in response to a moral event, you process a perception of harm, a perception of intent, some emotional response to that event, apply a cognitive description of what you saw, and form some motivation as an immediate response. All of this happens within the time span of an eye blink. All of these elements are experienced together, wrapped together. The emotional content infuses the cognitive description and the motivation.

Let's say that you witness an event that you feel is morally wrong. Your motivation will be the effect of wishing that this event stop, be stopped, or be avoided.

Our motivations attach to outcomes. We want to prevent harm, alleviate suffering, bring about good health outcomes, etc. As moral motivations, we fold emotional content into these outcomes, attaching a sense of personal commitment to them. If we are able to help bring about these desired outcomes, we feel **gratification**. If we are unable to bring about our desired outcomes, we are, obviously, not going to feel gratification.

Gratification is a feeling of pleasure at the satisfaction of a goal.

Of course, we all know that our hopes are not always realized and that our best efforts do not always pan out. Our attempts to do bring about desired outcomes sometimes fall short and we feel frustration. However, we also know that we sometimes consciously set aside our desires for gratification in favor of what we determine to be outcomes that take higher priority.

EXERCISE

When do you feel gratification? Imagine yourself in the future, feeling gratification at the accomplishment of your professional goals. What goals have been accomplished? How does this feel?

It was also noted in Chapter 1 that we can—and often should—exert executive control to modulate our intuitive reactions. We are prone to feeling some frustration when we put off outcomes that will gratify our moral feelings, though we often accept that it is wise to put off some gratification. Going to work might not be gratifying, but the trade-off (a paycheck) is for future outcomes that we deem to be worth the trade. This is delayed gratification. We also will surrender some gratification as exchange for another outcome that we rationally deem to be preferable—something like the "greater good" or adherence to an abstract principle under the justification of *doing the right thing*.

We are willing to accept this frustration as a trade-off if we see that we are delaying gratification for some outcome that is more desirable rationally. However, if we don't see the promise of a greater outcome, or the outcome never materializes despite our efforts, then the lack of gratification will produce moral dejection.

Delaying gratification can be stressful. We are typically creatures of the present. It takes effort to suspend some gratification for a future benefit. If that benefit isn't realized, the effort might seem wasted.

As we all know, our moral lives are far from direct and simple. In one event, you can perceive two people who intentionally cause harm to each other. Moral judgments can be formed against both. This is a case of conflict in which both parties are, to some extent, in the wrong.

When you face a moral conflict, your own emotional responses can pull you in different directions. You may know two people whose moral convictions are at odds with each other, and you wish to maintain friendly or working relationships with each. You may face a situation in which there are competing moral goods as possible outcomes. You may face a mix of emotional and rational responses to these options, recommending different options in different ways.

Sympathy, empathy, and compassion are responses to stress that arise when confronted with the pain and suffering of someone else. Sympathy and empathy seek gratification in escaping or avoiding this stress. Compassion is a willingness to be present with that suffering and be an instrument to its relief.

The kind of choices that an empathetic or compassionate moral agent wishes to make are ones that will alleviate the suffering of the other. Alleviating the patient's suffering will go a long way toward rising above one's own suffering. However, nurses and allied health professionals are limited in their ability to make these decisions. The decisions that most directly address patient suffering are treatment decisions. These are made by physicians, patients, or by the surrogates of patients. Other decisions are guided by protocols. There are good reasons to restrain the choices in this way. Still, this constraint against choice may produce feelings of helplessness or frustration in nursing and allied health professionals.

MORAL DEJECTION

This doesn't feel right.

Think of a situation in which you are able to do the right thing. You are gratified to see that good outcomes result from this action. This is a morally satisfying experience.

EXERCISE

Take a moment to identify some morally satisfying experiences. These can be small moments. Or, rather, we tend to take these for granted and so they seem small. Look at them closely now. Really, are these small?

This chapter will explore the experience of feeling morally dejected. These are the experiences in which you believe or wish that more could have been done.

In moral dejection, circumstances somehow do not allow for actions or outcomes that are fully morally satisfying. We experience moral dejection when we have in mind a right action or a good outcome but we cannot make it happen. Additionally, we experience moral dejection when we are in situations where we don't see the possibility of a good outcome, or we just don't know what the "right" action is no matter how hard we try to clarify it.

Moral dejection refers to an experience of frustration. As a moral agent, you recognize that you have choices to make and that there is moral weight to some of them. You recognize that you bear some responsibility for those choices, and you envision yourself as one who makes good moral choices. Sometimes, however, you face relatively tragic circumstances in which you cannot bring about the moral good you would otherwise wish to see. This frustration of your moral vision is dispiriting. This is moral dejection.

Moral dejection is a general term referring to a feeling of low spirits extending from a realization that one cannot bring about the moral good that one wishes.

In terms of moral agency, moral dejection arises when our ethical aspirations to be and do good meet circumstances that do not permit those dreams to come about. We may find that we are adding harm where we feel the intention to do no harm. We may find that we cannot promote good where we wish to promote it. Our hopes are frustrated and we meet with a measure of despair. It becomes difficult to offer a coherent narrative of value.

The challenge in moral dejection is to find value. There are two broad options: You either find value that you have been overlooking or you find actions or choices that position you to establish value.

A key to exploring moral dejection is found in the opening to the previous section. Moral dejection is a complex phenomenon. It involves a conflict with beliefs, motivations, hopes, and identity. The defining feature—that which agitates and exhausts—is emotion. It doesn't *feel* right. Chapter 1 touched on the manner in which emotions help to constitute our moral reactions. Emotions that arise within a moral reaction will be experienced differently depending, in part, on the motivation that accompanies them. A moral reaction will engage one's agency in varying ways. To suggest some of the variety in this engagement, we'll draw a comparison among sympathy, empathy, and compassion with respect to moral agency.

SYMPATHY, EMPATHY, AND COMPASSION

There is a current movement to present empathy as an emotional response that demonstrates care for patients and alleviates suffering. Compassion, on the other hand, is frequently presented as a source of fatigue. This book, and this chapter in particular, argue for a different view in which compassion is an interpersonal ethical skill. Rather than a source of fatigue is a potential source of moral satisfaction. As a skill, it compassion includes critical thinking and is a key element to professional integrity. As shown in earlier chapters, empathy is a mirrored response to the observation of suffering in someone else. By itself, it is an imperfect guide to moral action and also a source of stress.

Sympathy and empathy can build stress in you. The differences among sympathy, empathy, and compassion are not tightly defined. The presentation here represents a departure from some of the literature. This is due to the interest here in recognizing empathy as part of a mirrored response to suffering and in outlining a view of compassion as more than a reaction to stress.

Sympathy is a feeling that entails awareness of another as being capable of being harmed. It is a feeling of sorrow—even pity—directed toward another person for their real or potential suffering. Sympathy has also been described as *fellow-feeling*, a sense of emotional kinship with another. In both senses, sympathy has come to describe a fairly abstract connection with another person. You can be sympathetic toward someone and yet not empathetic. This would occur when you are sorrowful at the knowledge that another person is suffering and yet you do not feel a mirrored suffering of your own. This can also occur when you realize the possibility that someone else might suffer even though no such suffering is occurring right now.

Sympathy is more distant, more removed; whereas empathy is the taking in of something approximating someone else's pain. Of two people who witness the suffering of a third, the one who empathizes is able to say "I have an idea what you are going through" or "I had that same thing happen to me." The sympathizer would not be able to say this and could only offer a convention like "How awful for you. Is there anything I can do?" In other words, the sympathizer registers that someone is suffering, but is unable to connect with the type of suffering experienced by the other. The sympathizer is, perhaps, more willing to resort to platitudes (as found in the aptly named "sympathy cards"), expressions of pity, or even avoidance behaviors in response to someone else's pain.

The empathizer has some awareness of the other's pain—facilitated by mirrored pain and by comparable experience. Even for the empathizer, however, there may be an inability to see a suitable response to someone else's suffering. The mirrored pain that one feels might overwhelm or distract. Comparable experience will be limited in the insight it is able to deliver. The empathizer might be inspired to act as the empathizer would like the other to act were the tables reversed, but, without deeper insight into the sufferer's own experience, the empathizer might not choose an action to which the sufferer will best respond. What the sympathizer lacks is a shared space of emotion with the sufferer. What the empathizer lacks is the perspective of the sufferer. Relying on the experience of mirrored suffering, the empathizer operates from a point of bias (Prinz, 2011). The empathizer knows the suffering of the empathizer, not of the one who is the object of empathy. It is compassion that places the carer with the sufferer to attend and to listen.

There is a problem when we look to empathy combined with authentic presence as an intervention to make everything better. Empathy is a stress response. We mirror the suffering of another. With authentic presence, we are with someone who is suffering. We are with someone in their vulnerability and we become vulnerable in that space. There is suffering. Philosophically, we can observe that suffering is an ever-present facet of our lives. In health care, we know that suffering is ongoing. Even though we can see many patients get better, we will move on from those patients to the next patient whose suffering needs attention. No matter the perspective, suffering will always be encountered. Empathy responds to suffering as a problem to be addressed or escaped. Yet the environment of health care is one of a continuous series of individuals who suffer. If we feel empathy for all these individuals, then the mirrored suffering we feel never abates. If we think that empathy and authentic presence are to make everything magically better, then we might wonder what we're doing wrong.

Let's examine some ways in which nurses experience moral dejection: moral distress, moral residue, and what is commonly labeled compassion fatigue. These are cited as factors in burnout, stress, and cynicism.

MORAL DISTRESS

Moral distress is a response to a situation in which there is a conflict between your personal moral convictions and the expectations that other people have for you. When those expectations are orders or regulations that you must follow, there is conflict between what you are

Moral distress describes the condition in which external constraints prevent you from doing the right thing.

told to do and what you believe is the right thing to do. The conflict is particularly acute when you believe that the orders you are given are morally wrong (Humphries & Woods, 2016; Jameton, 2017).

The suffering you encounter in the health-care environment is stressful by itself. When you are asked to perform an act that you find morally offensive, the stress compounds. For the most part, it is likely that you will often feel that your work aligns with your moral beliefs. The conflict of moral distress arises as an exception to your typical routine. The order that conflicts with your beliefs stands out; it demands attention. There is an incompatibility between what you are told to do and what you want to do (Jameton, 2017; Schluter, Winch, Holzhauser, & Henderson, 2008).

The conflict will often involve your own personal beliefs on the administrative level. This is where you draw boundaries, judging certain actions or behaviors as always wrong or always right. We can draw these administrative lines around issues that are sources of considerable moral controversy. You are already familiar with several of these. We can also draw administrative lines around issues pertaining to medical futility and other issues in bioethics.

CLINICAL MORALITY VERSUS PERSONAL MORALITY

The professional role will condition you to respond in certain ways to certain situations. This is a practical consequence of doing the job. This professional conditioning begins as a matter of training the *hand* to follow rules, regulations, protocols, procedures. In time, following these becomes somewhat instinctive—a training of the *heart* while on the job.

In moral distress, you are aware of the conflict as you are made to act in the clinical setting. Feeling the emotional effects of this conflict, you might wonder, *What have I done?* after you leave the clinical setting. The way you acted was instinctive, conditioned. It is when you reflect on this in a different setting, in a different social role, that you might wonder about your actions. Or, more personally, you wonder about the instinctive nature of those actions. You might begin to wonder about who you have become such that you could act like this.

Where this is conflict between clinical morality and personal morality, your personal beliefs can be deeply offended. This conflict is persistent so that you feel that your work always requires you to act this way. The effect is that this conflict—your job—is challenging who you are as a person, as a moral agent.

Issues where people might experience moral distress are often issues in which people have firmly made up their minds. Open-ended discourse about these issues can be hard to come by. People are often so invested in their administrative beliefs about these issues that they seek to promote or defend their beliefs rather than critically examine them alongside alternative views (Burston & Tuckett, 2013).

EXERCISE

Identify some of the controversial issues that might give rise to conflicts that result in feelings of moral distress. Discuss and compare your list with the lists compiled by other students.

The public treatment of controversial issues tends to reduce the views to two sides, pro and con. In reality, controversies have many sides and there are many differing opinions. Because we refrain from sharing these opinions in open discourse, we miss the diversity of perspectives. Controversies that restrict views in this way and do not admit of reasonable discourse are sources of stress. This stress can have an entertainment factor in public media and it can be a motivating factor in the political arena. When these controversies enter into your professional life and impede your view of your own pursuit of professional integrity, they become sources of personal stress.

ADDRESSING MORAL DISTRESS

In politics and in public life we poorly equip ourselves to resolve moral controversy. We settle for an *us versus them* attitude. In your professional life, *us versus them* gets in the way of effective collaboration and can negatively impact patient outcomes and a culture of safety. There is a need, then, for ethical skills to address moral distress when it arises.

In the heart/hand/head model, moral distress can be seen as a conflict between heart and hand. What the heart wants to do is in conflict with what the hand has been ordered to do. The head's task is to mediate between your feelings and the task that is given to you. The ethical skill you need to employ is a critical examination of the administrative-level beliefs that are drawing hard lines and causing you to see conflict.

The point of focus is on your administrative-level beliefs. Think about what you believe. Try to engage this examination of beliefs without falling into an *us versus them* mentality. Identify that part of what you have been told to do that is in conflict with your beliefs. Can you find any value in the principles behind that order? Is it possible to see that your orders are consistent with autonomy, beneficence, nonmaleficence, or justice? Is it possible to use the categorical imperative to show that your orders are morally permissible? This conflict puts you in position to review your moral beliefs. Test your own beliefs in the same way.

EXERCISE

Identify a belief you have about a moral controversy. Use the administrative-level assessment part of the Ethical Assessment Model to explore views that differ from yours. What insight are you able to gain by doing this?

If this examination of beliefs does not help you to find a way to resolve the conflict, then look for an appropriate forum in which to express your concerns and ask for clarification. Keep your mind open and listen carefully to any defense that is offered for the orders that have been given to you. Do what you can to find your voice in this issue. Can you advocate for yourself? Can you find an advocate who can help make sure that your perspective is considered?

Above all, make certain that you maintain focus on the interpersonal level. Are you taking a stand for the patient or are you taking a stand for an issue? Be careful not to confuse the two. Is your distress distracting you from a willingness to compassionately attend to your patient?

Compassion should be employed in thinking about beliefs and talking about the issue. Try to see the people behind the orders with which you disagree. Humanizing them can help keep you from framing the issue as *us versus them* When seeking your voice as you talk about this issue, remember to compassionately listen as well. If the issue is hard for you it might also be hard for someone else. Listening open ears and opens minds. As you are compassionate, so you establish the chance for others to reciprocate by listening compassionately to you. You don't have to appeal to someone else's sense of empathy by declaring how much you have suffered. It might be enough to reach out and offer a listening ear and pledge to compassionately work through the problem.

Compassion is especially needed for all involved when a decision must be made to withhold or withdraw treatment from an end-stage patient. Nobody wants to make a decision that results in death. When it comes to ending futile care, it's important to recognize that, while the decision about treatment results in death, it does not cause death.

MORAL RESIDUE

Moral Residue is the product of an ethical dilemma. Whereas moral distress mainly involves administrative-level beliefs, moral residue is the product of facing strategic-level decisions that don't allow us to act to effectively bring about all the results we would like to see.

"When you get to a fork in the road, take it." Attributed to baseball icon Yogi Berra, this possibly apocryphal quote does well to capture the conflict we feel when we face an ethical dilemma. We face a choice, like a fork in the road. Both are ways to a desirable destination. Each destination has features that the other lacks. Each destination has some appeal, but neither one is so superior to the other that it makes the other destination seem like a poor choice. We want what both destinations offer, but we have to choose. Choosing one means turning away from the other. We know that a choice has to be made, but, even facing the choice, we already begin to feel some regret that we can't have it all. We want to take the fork, not just one of the tines.

An **ethical dilemma** is a situation in which different courses of action each present the appeal of producing some moral good. There isn't any course of action available that would produce all possible moral good. Choosing one action, then, means that some moral good will not be brought about. That choice can bring about feelings of guilt or regret for the good that could not be achieved.

There are specific features of an ethical dilemma: As a moral agent, you face a choice between two or more options. Each of these options can be seen as morally permissible or even obligatory. Each option stands to produce some outcome that is morally good. However, the options available do not promise to lead to the same good outcomes. While each should produce some good, none is able to produce all of the good that the other options can produce. This means that you cannot make a choice that will produce all the moral good that the options collectively cover. Something has to be left behind. No matter what choice you make, your choice means that you will decide not to act to bring about some good.

Moral residue arises in the wake of making a choice in an ethical dilemma. The choice made is to bring about a certain good result. But making that choice means turning away from other good results that could have been brought about if other options had been chosen. Moral residue is the regret felt at the sacrifice of other options. Yes, some good has been done, but what about the good that could have been done?

It might seem that there is a problem of proportion in feeling moral residue. A choice made in an ethical dilemma represents the choice to bring about good. Yet, we feel the choice to be agonizing because, as moral agents, we are more drawn to the good that must be sacrificed

Moral residue is a feeling of regret or guilt the extends from participating in an ethical dilemma.

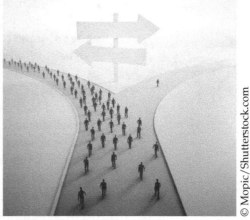

Figure 7.1

An **ethical dilemma** is a choice of action, the options of which each offer some good. Choosing one option means choosing against some other possible good. An ethical dilemma is symmetrical if the available options promise relatively equal degrees of good. In an asymmetrical dilemma, there is one option that is clearly superior to the others. Still, some good is left unattained by choosing this better option.

in the options we don't choose. The foundational concept in health-care ethics is *first do no harm*. We are quick to notice harm, and we are often more upset at the prospect of harm than we are gratified at the prospect of doing good. The phenomenon of moral residue tends to bear out this idea that we focus more on allowing harm than we do at facilitating good. Though we are able to do some good in an ethical dilemma, it is the good not done and the harm that might accrue as a result that gnaws at our consciences. We can feel remorse or guilt.

The various forms of moral dejection are reactions and always depend in part on the emotional reactions of the people involved. These reactions depend on the individuals. They also can be shaped by particular elements that are relative to the choices presented in the dilemma. As a rule, for instance, moral residue will be stronger and more challenging in situations that involve considerable suffering or risk of death. The higher the stakes, the harder the choice.

The choice in an ethical dilemma also will be more difficult as the choices appear to be equally compelling. Such a condition is called a *symmetrical dilemma*. This is a condition in which at least two options in a dilemma promise good results that are relatively equal in value or importance. The argument for one option is just as strong as for another. It is hard to choose and the choice is more agonizing. In contrast, an *asymmetrical dilemma* presents one option that has clear advantages over other options. There can still be residue for the good left undone, but there might be some solace in that the right course of action was rather clear to choose.

You can be affected with moral residue even if you are not the moral agent who bears the responsibility for making the choice. Treatment decisions concerning a patient, for example, are typically made by the patient, the physician and possibly by the patient's family or surrogate. Nurses and allied health professionals often do not have a say in these decisions. But you are a moral agent, and you are involved in the patient's care. As a moral agent you might be inclined to think along with the decision-making process. Your empathy and your compassion might place you in the difficulty of the situation. You also have a stake in this choice because your orders will extend from whatever decision is made. Even though you are on the periphery of the decision-making, you still can be prone to experiencing moral residue.

The choice between options is a strategic-level decision. In a dilemma, you will have to weigh the potential outcomes from the options available. Utilitarian thinking provides a way to draw a comparison between these options. Carefully scrutinize these options and make your best choice. Utilitarian thinking approach can help provide strategic guidance in making this choice.

Once a choice has been made—even a choice that has been strategically identified as the one that is the best available—there is still the possibility of experiencing moral residue. How do you respond to moral residue, whether or not you have a choice to make in the dilemma? How do you prepare for the remorse, the guilt?

Before you can weigh options, you first need to recognize them. The perception of the options available to us can be limited by the outcomes we are able, or allow ourselves, to see. The expectations we carry into a situation—possibly influenced by organizational and personal administrative-level beliefs—can serve to limit our view of potential options. As you look at this situation, identify your own personal administrative-level beliefs.

When other people are involved in the decision-making, try to take note of the options that they see. Can you identify the administrative-level beliefs that are driving people in this situation who have a stake in this decision? Try to be open to understanding the perspective these people carry into making this decision.

Recognize that the decision that is made sets the course forward. Once made, this decision is what will be followed. Your willingness to align with this decision is needed. If others had the responsibility for making this decision, compassionately recognize the challenges they had to face in making this choice. If you feel moral residue, remember that this is an effect of the ethical dilemma more than it is a product of the decision itself. Recognize that if you feel moral residue others likely feel it too. Your compassion toward them can help them cope with the remorse they feel. Reaching out to others in this way can have the reciprocal effect of helping ease any remorse that you feel as well (Barlow, Hargreaves, & Gillibrand, 2018).

"COMPASSION FATIGUE" AND COMPASSION SATISFACTION

Literature abounds on the phenomenon of compassion fatigue. What is described is an experience of feeling depleted, a professionally crippling loss of the capacity to care for those who suffer. The source of this depletion is the exposure to suffering. There is so much demand in caring for those who suffer that one's reserves become exhausted, producing this form of moral dejection. Compassion is sometimes said to be that which leads to this dejection. One only has so much to give, it seems. Once your limit is reached, compassion has drained you.

While the experience of fatigue is real, compassion is not the source. Part of the problem with the literature is that the name **"compassion fatigue"** came to be applied without a careful investigation into the nature of compassion. Remember that there is a difference between empathy—a moral reaction—and compassion—an ethical skill. The source of fatigue is empathy and not compassion.

Empathy associates with a desire to fix what is wrong—to bring a stressful situation to resolution. When a neat solution to tidiness is not presented, stress further compounds. All of these are the ingredients for so-called compassion fatigue. Compassion, though, isn't the problem.

Compassion fatigue is a term used to describe a feeling of exhaustion or indifference due to prior excessive feelings of empathy (perhaps better understood as empathy fatigue).

Empathy fatigue is a feeling of exhaustion or indifference due to prior excessive feelings of empathy (more commonly referred to as compassion fatigue).

This form of moral dejection is better termed **empathy fatigue**. Empathy can be is fatiguing because there is a lack of adequate redress of your own suffering that is felt in response to the suffering of someone else.

Compassion, with its combination of intense imaginative engagement, transactional listening, humility, and critical thinking, presents certain advantages. It is, first of all, a distraction from your own suffering because you are attending primarily to the suffering of the other. In listening to someone else, you give the other the assurance that you are present and, thereby, affirm that person's humanity and worth. This interpersonal connection has some facility to reduce suffering in the other and in you. Compassion also is better suited to difficult situations because you are better able to move within ambiguity.

Compassion is a nourishing cycle. We feed others as we act compassionately toward them. In turn, we are fed when others act compassionately toward us and as we act compassionately. The skill is driven by willingness to care for, and pay attention to, the patient as a person who has an interest in a significant life. Through this willingness, one reaches out to care as the patient reaches out to be cared for. In this meeting of you and your patient—one who cares and one who is cared for—there is reciprocal affirmation. Your willing attention demonstrates that you believe that your patient is a person who matters. As you recognize your patient in this way, you realize the worth of reaching out. The compassionate connection itself is a gesture of care. Compassion doesn't cure all ills, but it adds value merely by being present.

Empathy, meanwhile, motivates reactions that are biased to the mirrored suffering that one feels. You reach out to another, not based on your affirmation of the person, but based on how you transpose your feelings onto the other person. Empathy can be consistent with compassionate care, but it is not by itself a reliable means to witness another person's suffering. When there is this mismatch, there can be misunderstanding or clumsy expressions of care. Suffering persists. It can even compound (Buchanan, Bagley, Stansfield, & Preston, 2012; Loggia, Mogil, & Catherine, 2008). As empathy fails to discharge suffering, the suffering builds and this can be fatiguing.

In terms of care, the attention-giving that is part of the skill of compassion enables you to listen to the narrative of your patient and draw a more nuanced view of your patient's needs. Your capacity to provide care is enhanced. Here, again, your patient potentially benefits from your compassionate care. Moreover, again, you gain the sense of worth in reaching out with compassion.

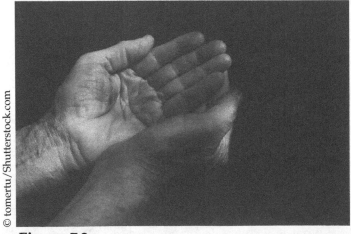

© tomertu/Shutterstock.com

Figure 7.2

Where there is compassion, there are benefits in enhanced care and in the experience of interpersonal connection. Compassionate connection brings an awareness of worth of both the other person and you. In this way, compassion feeds. Fatigue does not result from being compassionate toward others. It results when you are in need of compassion.

Patients in their suffering and vulnerability might invite you in. When they do they are looking for someone who is trustworthy, someone who will pay attention to them and see them as a person. Such patients feel reduced by their condition. They feel discredited. They yearn for someone who will acknowledge them as people who matter.

Empathy is a moral reaction. It is the mirroring of your observation of the suffering of others. Empathy produces suffering in you. Your response to this suffering can be agential or nonagential. In nonagential empathy, you recognize no capacity to act on behalf of the one who suffers. The suffering generated by seeing someone who is actively suffering remains with you.

In agential actions that extend from empathy, you are motivated to do something for the one who suffers. Your action is guided by your own mirrored suffering. You put yourself in the other person's place and base your action on what you would want. There are additional problems with empathy as motivation for action. As seen in Chapter 3, empathy biases our view of moral situations. It can be unfairly oriented to those we regard as belonging to one's in-group, and it can discourage us from acting on behalf of those for whom we feel some level of distaste (Decety & Cowell, 2015; Prinz, 2011).

Whether agential or nonagential in relation to action, empathy builds suffering but does not provide an effective means of discharging the suffering. If you don't channel empathy through compassion, it can become a source of stress. Too much empathy without compassion sets the condition under which suffering builds to a level where it becomes stressful or leads to burnout. Fatigue results. The source of fatigue is empathy, not compassion.

EXERCISE

If compassion fatigue is a misleading term, then consider what *compassion satisfaction* might mean. Offer your own description of what compassion does for us as we encounter those who suffer. Define compassion satisfaction.

Emmanuel Levinas offered a view of what he termed *useless suffering*. This kind of suffering has two conditions: (1) This is "unassumable". You want to completely reject this. You do not want to this to happen to you. You might think, *This is not why I got into nursing* or *This is not how I want to see myself.* It is unbearable, and yet it cannot be avoided or rejected. (2) The second condition is passivity. What you want to reject cannot be rejected. This unassumable event is happening to you and you cannot make this go away. Whatever agency you have, you are unable to escape, remove, or otherwise solve the problem posed by your suffering. It overwhelms. The situation that morally discourages you isn't going to magically change to a happily ever after moral outcome (Lévinas, 1998).

Andres has been living with Amyotrophic Lateral Sclerosis (ALS). His illness is unassumable. He doesn't want this. With everything he has, he wishes he didn't have to deal with this. But he has no choice, no ability to just make this go away. ALS will disable him. This will make him other than the person he aspires to be. This will cause his death.

Clinically, there are things we can do to address the causes and symptoms of conditions that bring a patient to suffer. But other aspects of the patient's suffering—the loss of social identity, stigma, feeling a burden to others, hopelessness—cannot be physically treated. Andres needs medical care. This medical care cannot cure his ALS, nor can medical treatments fix these aspects of his suffering.

Levinas applies the word *useless* to this type of suffering. The experience of suffering is so personal to the patient. It is experienced as an unwarranted assault on the person. The assault is such that the person can feel utterly thrown out of a normal life. This suffering is useless to the patient's view of what a normal life is and ought to be. Of course, not all patients are Andres. Many patients face good outcomes and the restoration of a normal life. In the course of illness, though, many patients will feel their suffering to be unassumable yet imposed on them nonetheless. Many patients will strive to make sense of their suffering as they recover. But in the midst, they are prone to experience their suffering as useless.

Unassumable suffering cannot be taken away. When we feel empathy for someone like Andres, we experience a form of mirrored suffering. This is an instinctive imagining of what it would be like in Andres' place. Andres doesn't want his suffering and, feeling empathy, neither do we. For us, suffering is a problem to be fixed or evaded. We imagine ourselves in Andres' place and try to find some way to help Andres escape the problem. However, we cannot fix this aspect of his suffering. Further, because we don't have Andres' experience, we cannot know what this is like for him. Empathy provides us a way to imagine ourselves in his place, but this cannot give us any confidence that we know what it is like for him. We only know the suffering we feel and the motivation we have to relieve him from his burden. Through empathy, we can try to demonstrate to Andres that we care about him, that we feel for him. Empathy, by itself, doesn't show us what Andres needs from us.

Only Andres can show us what he needs. Empathy can draw us toward Andres as an object of concern. At this point, Andres is still held at a distance as we view him through the lens of the suffering we feel and imagine. Now, if we have the willingness, we can open to Andres' own narrative of his suffering. This is compassion. Levinas describes this an *inter*-human connection in which one person reaches out for help and someone else reaches out to help.

Empathy is a source of stress. It is your felt response to someone else's suffering. Empathy does not offer a solution. Compassion empowers. As you are willing to open to the patient's narrative of the experience of suffering, you establish an interhuman connection that, in itself, acknowledges the patient as someone who matters. You are also positioned to better understand what you can do to better care for this patient. However, even at this level of establishing this connection, you have reached out and offered the patient acknowledgment that you see the person and not just the suffering.

TAKEAWAY

Moral dejection deflates. It brings you low. Ethics isn't always easy. We turn our attention to ethics, in fact, when things get hard. Dejection is a cost of being morally aware.

However, there is hope. Doing ethics and making moral choices can be demanding, but you can meet those demands. You can't avoid all circumstances that can lead to moral dejection, but there are things you can do.

You can engage ethical thinking in such a way as to make the best choices you can. Yet, you will still encounter situations in which your administrative-level beliefs do not initially align with those of others. There will still be ethical dilemmas that admit of no ideal solution. In your professional career, you will feel empathy for many people who suffer, and you will face the burden of the mirrored suffering that builds in you.

Ethical assessment can help you navigate these challenges. The Ethical Assessment Model won't deliver you to perfect solutions, but it can help you to gain perspective, to set your priorities, to build your integrity, and to find a way to move in a difficult landscape.

CASE STUDIES

CASE STUDY 7.1—MORAL DISTRESS

Chloe is a 16-year-old female. She is in the ICU, sedated, and intubated. She is experiencing multisystem organ failure due to septicemia. She has a poor prognosis. Her parents want to spare her any more suffering and make the decision to withdraw her from life support.

(Continued)

Alec has been Chloe's nurse since admission to the ICU. Alec thinks that, given enough time, Chloe can respond to treatment. He is tempted to say something to the parents, but he feels it's not his place. Alec knows that Chloe's parents are already grieving their daughter. He still feels that they are not making a good decision.

How should Alec respond to his moral distress? Use the Ethical Assessment Model to evaluate the options available to Alec. Use this model to assess the decision made by Chloe's parents.

CASE STUDY 7.2—BURIDAN'S CHOICE

Buridan is a 77-year-old male, suffering from renal carcinoma. He faces a choice between two treatment options. He can opt for a surgical procedure or a research trial. Buridan lives at home with his wife, Pearl. Pearl has severe dementia, and Buridan is her primary caregiver.

Buridan is alone in the office of his oncologist, Dr. Antov. He is talking with Dr. Antov's nurse, Yolanda. Buridan likes the surgical option because it seems tried and true. "You just go in and get it, right?" But, at the same time, he is disturbed by the time he will have to spend in the hospital and the recovery period after. "I have to be there for Pearl." He asks Yolanda to explain the research drug trial again. Finally, Buridan sighs and says, "I think that will be best." Yolanda reads him through the consent form and obtains his signatures.

Six months later, Dr. Antov gives Buridan the sad news that a CT scan shows that his tumor has grown 50% beyond the baseline scan from when he entered the trial. MRI results indicate metastases in the lungs and his brain. Because of the size of the growth of the tumor, Buridan is now excluded from this research trial. Because of the metastases, surgery is no longer an option for him.

Later that day, Yolanda expresses to Dr. Antov her regret about Buridan. She can't help but think that Buridan might have had a better outcome if he had chosen the surgical option six months ago. She knows that the decision was his and that she had no say in it at all. But she thinks of his wife. She thinks of what could have been. If only . . .

Imagine that Yolanda uses the Ethical Assessment Model. Using this, how will she review her own actions and the choice made by Buridan?

CASE STUDY 7.3—EMPATHY FATIGUE

Melina is waiting at the Perk 'n' Pour coffee shop. She's been waiting nearly a half hour for her friend and coworker Aubrey. Melina is nearly finished with her coffee when Aubrey rushes into the shop. She is effusively apologetic. She was running behind and couldn't let Melina know because her phone battery is drained and she can't find her charger. Melina responds that this isn't like Aubrey—or, rather, wasn't until recently. "What's going on?"

Aubrey and Melina work together in an ICU unit. Today, Aubrey was assigned to a patient who died four hours after she came on shift. She never knew the patient, but she listened to the stories the family had to tell about him. The stories were so eloquent and beautiful. "They loved this man so much," Aubrey says. "And I could picture him. I swear, the descriptions they gave of him reminded me so much of my grandfather. I could picture this man. I really could. I never met him. But I feel like I know him. I almost feel like I lost someone today." Aubrey further explains that this isn't the first time. She's lost patients before. She's seen families devastated by loss. More and more, her heart aches with each loss. She feels so badly for all these people. "I feel like I go to work every day to get my heart broken."

What advice can Melina give? Should Melina give any advice at all? Use the Ethical Assessment Model to explore what Melina can do to respond to Aubrey's suffering.

REFERENCES

AHA Hospital Statistics. (2018). *Fast facts on U.S. Hospitals.* Chicago, IL: AHA Resource Center. Retrieved from https://www.aha.org/statistics/fast-facts-us-hospitals

Barlow, N. A., Hargreaves, J., & Gillibrand, W. P. (2018). Nurses' contributions to the resolution of ethical dilemmas in practice. *Nursing Ethics, 25*(2), 230–242.

Buchanan, T. W, Bagley, S. L., Stansfield, R. B., & Preston, S. D. (2012). The empathic, physiological resonance of stress. *Social Neuroscience, 7*(2), 191–201.

Burston, A. S., & Tuckett, A. G. (2013). Moral distress in nursing: contributing factors, outcomes and interventions. *Nursing Ethics, 20*(3), 312–324.

Decety, J., & Cowell, J. M. (2015). 17 The equivocal relationship between morality and empathy. *The Moral Brain: A Multidisciplinary Perspective,* 279.

Humphries, A., & Woods, M. (2016). A study of nurses' ethical climate perceptions: Compromising in an uncompromising environment. *Nursing Ethics, 23*(3), 265–276.

Jameton, A. (2017). What moral distress in nursing history could suggest about the future of health care. *AMA Journal of Ethics, 19*(6), 617–628.

Lévinas, E. (1998). *Entre Nous: On thinking-of-the-other.* London: Athlone Press.

Loggia, M. L., Mogil, J. S., & Catherine, B. M. (2008). Empathy hurts: Compassion for another increases both sensory and affective components of pain perception. *Pain, 136,* 168–176.

Maiden, J., Georges, J. M., & Connelly, C. D. (2011). Moral distress, compassion fatigue, and perceptions about medication errors in certified critical care nurses. *Dimensions of Critical Care Nursing, 30*(6), 339–345.

Prinz, J. (2011). Is empathy necessary for morality. *Empathy: Philosophical and Psychological Perspectives, 1,* 211–229.

Schluter, J., Winch, S., Holzhauser, K., & Henderson, A. (2008). Nurses' moral sensitivity and hospital ethical climate: A literature review. *Nursing Ethics, 15*(3), 304–321.

U.S. Bureau of Labor Statistics. (2018a). *Occupational employment and wages, May 2017: 29-1071 physician assistants.* NE Washington, D.C.: U.S. Bureau of Labor Statistics. Retrieved from https://www.bls.gov/oes/current/oes291071.htm

U.S. Bureau of Labor Statistics. (2018b). *Occupational employment and wages, May 2017: 29-1122 occupational therapists.* NE Washington, D.C.: U.S. Bureau of Labor Statistics. Retrieved from https://www.bls.gov/oes/current/oes291122.htm

U.S. Bureau of Labor Statistics. (2018c). *Occupational employment and wages, May 2017: 29-1123 physical therapists.* NE Washington, D.C.: U.S. Bureau of Labor Statistics. Retrieved from https://www.bls.gov/oes/current/oes291123.htm

U.S. Bureau of Labor Statistics. (2018d). *Occupational employment and wages, May 2017: 29-1126 respiratory therapists.* NE Washington, D.C.: U.S. Bureau of Labor Statistics. Retrieved from https://www.bls.gov/oes/current/oes291126.htm

U.S. Bureau of Labor Statistics. (2018e). *Occupational employment and wages, May 2017: 29-1141 registered nurses.* NE Washington, D.C.: U.S. Bureau of Labor Statistics. Retrieved from https://www.bls.gov/oes/current/oes291141.htm

U.S. Bureau of Labor Statistics. (2018f). *Occupational employment and wages, May 2017: 29-1171 nurse practitioners.* NE Washington, D.C.: U.S. Bureau of Labor Statistics. Retrieved from https://www.bls.gov/oes/current/oes291171.htm

U.S. Bureau of Labor Statistics. (2018g). *Occupational Employment and Wages, May 2017: 31-1014 nursing assistants.* NE Washington, D.C.: U.S. Bureau of Labor Statistics. Retrieved from https://www.bls.gov/oes/current/oes311014.htm

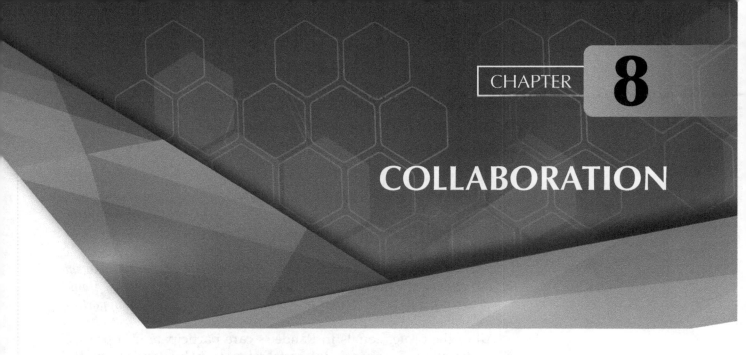

CHAPTER 8

COLLABORATION

OBJECTIVES

After completing this chapter, you will be able to . . .

1. Refine your awareness of the significance of communication by placing it in the context of collaboration.

2. Integrate the virtues of advocacy into an examination of collaboration.

3. Process the importance of harmony in a healthcare environment and apply its principles to handoff and other forms of communication.

4. Scrutinize the problems and causes of horizontal and vertical violence.

5. Apply the Ethical Assessment Model to chapter exercises and to real-life scenarios.

KEY TERM

- Negative capability

Box 8.1 Responsibilities to the Profession 13

The dietetics practitioner presents reliable and substantiated information and interprets controversial information without personal bias, recognizing that legitimate differences of opinion exist (Edge et al., 2009)

INTRODUCTION

Collaboration is a process. It is a shared effort to join in a multidisciplinary team to bring healthcare to individuals and populations who are in need.

Randee is a nine-year old fourth grader who presents with asthmatic symptoms in class. Her teacher takes her to the school nurse. The nurse calls for an ambulance. The paramedics take her to the emergency department (ED) at the local hospital. A medical team in the ED treats her and stabilizes her. A physician writes an order for admission and Randee is transferred to the pediatric floor. Randee sees a new doctor on the pediatric floor. By now she has also encountered several nurses, a respiratory therapist, medical transport personnel, and several other professionals—all involved in supporting Randee's care.

All of the professionals in Randee's care participate in a process of collaboration. Everyone's interest serves to help Randee breathe again. Within a matter of hours, many people report on Randee's case. There are many intersections in which various professionals, with their particular expertise and experience, offer their part in the continuum of Randee's care. Their reporting needs to be consistent, providing the right information in a way in which other professionals expect to find it.

In reporting, we say what is known. There is also an element of the unknown. The patient might still be in the diagnostic phase and reporting keeps track of what comes to light. Once diagnosed, reporting keeps track of the developing outcome.

COMMUNICATION

In Chapter 6, communication was identified as a means to avoid errors and promote a culture of safety. We now further identify communication as essential to the process of collaboration. Effective communication is, therefore, essential to the goals of healthcare as a whole. There needs to be an exchange of ideas, knowledge, observations, concerns, and feelings. The patient needs the attention of an entire healthcare team, acting together for successful outcomes. It is communication that enables the team to function for the good of the patient.

Communication is the framework of healthcare. Care is very coordinated and collaboration is essential to that coordination. Advocacy involves a call for aid and a response. This works within a healthcare team as a coordinated response to that call. Without effective communication, there is no coordination. The team has to communicate in order to coordinate care. Communication is the lifeblood of collaboration.

An established chain of communication facilitates continuity of care. Veracity requires that you offer complete and accurate reporting.

On the level of administrative assessment, accurate and complete reporting serves nonmaleficence. Report so as to do no harm.

If you think of yourself as an individual agent, nonmaleficence can require little more than refraining from causing harm. It grows more complicated when your agency is part of a team effort to deliver care. Now, you not only have the responsibility to refrain from actions that cause harm, you also need to contribute to the team's overall understanding of the patient's case so no one else causes harm. You also need information from other members of the team, so that you better understand how to keep your patient from harm.

Communication has a flow. It moves as each person in the chain contributes information. Standards for reporting help to ensure the consistency of the communication process, but it remains complex and dynamic. The process does not just rely on healthcare professionals. The participation of patients and family members is also needed.

VIRTUES OF COLLABORATION

If you do your job in healthcare, you are collaborating. Collaboration is part of your professional integrity. The wholeness of your integrity is itself a part of the wholeness of a patient's healthcare team. As you perform your role responsibly, the team is better positioned to treat the patient with safe and appropriate care.

Because collaboration is part of a healthcare team's response to a patient's call for aid, we can see that the virtues of being a patient advocate apply also to effective collaboration.

TRUST IN COLLABORATION

Trustworthiness in healthcare is an ethical skill of meeting the expectations of your professional role with responsibility and accountability. Responsibility is internally oriented, applying to your own devotion to upholding the expectations of your professional role. Being accountable has an external orientation, applying to the way in which you stand behind your performance in your role and hold your work out publicly as a demonstration of how well you meet expectations. Responsibility is what you feel and accountability is what you show.

In collaboration each person in the healthcare team needs to trust that other members will reliably perform their tasks, lend their expertise, and present the facts in communication (McCabe & Sambrook, 2014). The stakes can be high. Failures in upholding the expectations of one's role, including failures in communication, can lead to harm. Holding yourself accountable demonstrates your trustworthiness.

Trustworthiness needs to be sustainable in order for it to be effective. Responsibility is a continuing devotion to your role. You need to develop the pattern of reliability so that coworkers know what to expect from you. Accountability shows up as coworkers not only expect you to fulfill the tasks of your role but also to have the quality of a dedicated professional. Trusting you in this way, your coworkers might be less inclined to react to a mistake of yours as a condemnation of your skills or responsibility.

There is something indescribable about trustworthiness. While job duties can be detailed, professional responsibility cannot be broken down into a list. We can see when people perform their tasks, but this observation is somewhat different from seeing that someone has brought accountability into the performance of job duties. There is no protocol for integrity, and yet some will say that they know it when they see it.

EXERCISE

Think about the traits you want to see in a coworker. How can you tell when you work with someone who is responsible and trustworthy?

Clinical systems are designed to foster trust. There are strategic guides that ensure consistency of communication and reporting standards. For the most part, this means that you can trust a coworker that you don't know. You share in the same outcomes and plan of care for a given patient. You are accountable to the same procedures. This enables a working level of trust.

Trust depends on people doing more than reporting. It's possible to fulfill the technical aspects of a job while not doing so with integrity. There has to be a willingness to give your effort to the tasks of the job. The strategic level of accomplishing tasks needs to be complemented by the interpersonal level of acting with compassionate responsibility for the wellbeing of your patients and coworkers.

Remember your oath and code. Professional integrity doesn't merely ask you perform the tasks that are assigned to you. Integrity asks for your commitment to your role. Take on the role, presenting it as an image of who you are. Hold the responsibility to show your dedication to your patients and to your profession. Demonstrate your accountability to your role, not merely to your assigned tasks. Show your trustworthiness through who you are as a professional.

EXERCISE

Personalities sometimes clash. You will not get along with all of your coworkers. To what extent does your friendship with someone impact your trust for that person?

VERACITY

Veracity in communication is an important element in demonstrating trustworthiness. Accuracy and being forthcoming are necessary skills. Withholding or embellishing information are crucial aspects of veracity. As you report, you speak to what you have observed.

Reporting standards focus on what is known, such as a patient's history. The history tells the patient's medical course. This helps to direct care and avoid putting the patient at risk. At the beginning of a shift, in taking a report, you are about to gather everything that is known about a patient. At this moment, you are at a threshold. You've been given the known. You are about to enter the unknown.

We don't know how a patient will respond to treatment. We don't know each patient as a person. We don't know what is going to happen from moment to moment. There is also an element of veracity in mystery.

Veracity entails dedication to speaking the truth. Medical practice is evidence based. As you report, you provide the evidence without bias or ornamentation. Your report, however, can only speak to part of the experience of providing care.

Truth unfolds. The patient's history is given to you as a snapshot of what has been. Because the patient remains in care, it is clear that this medical

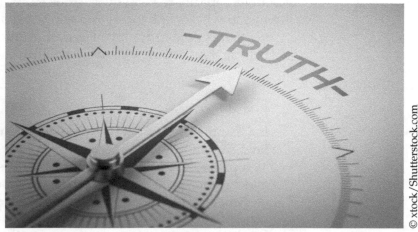

Figure 8.1

history has not come to a close. It continues to declare. The history you have been given is a work in progress. You have the task of recording the patient's history as it unfolds under your care. Veracity includes your dedication to this task.

Veracity isn't only about speaking truth. It also includes your comportment toward the evidence that will emerge. Veracity, as devotion to truth, requires the *negative capability* to acknowledge what is not known and to be open to whatever truth emerges.

Holding negative capability, you do not sit in utter unknowing. The history of a patient has been declared. This history can, and should, enable you to anticipate the future of this patient's medical trajectory. But there is a difference between anticipation and expectation. To expect is to believe that you know what will or what should happen. To anticipate is to believe that something is likely to happen.

Negative capability is an attitude in which one is able to surrender a need to be fully in control and to be certain about is happening and will happen. It is the capacity to face uncertainty and still function.

Negative capability has application as an interpersonal skill. The capacity to acknowledge truth as it spontaneously unfolds leads to effective action. The lack of veracity is a lack of compassion. Have the patience and humility to be attentive.

Embracing negative capability means having the willingness to attend to your patient. This interpersonal connection enables you to affirm your patient as a person. It further means attending to your patient without assumptions. Have the willingness to be open to your patient's narrative, using this to learn better about your patient's needs. Have the willingness to witness your patient's condition as it declares itself. Negative capability can improve your care and position you to respond to complications as they arise.

When things get stressful, focus on what is known. Be careful not to confuse what you see with what you want to see. Holding your willingness to attend to your patient, observe the facts and report them as accurately as you can. Stress might inhibit some of your ability to report accurately. Do your best and remember where your focus needs to be.

Negative capability is not easy. It requires a measure of humility and a capacity to be in mystery. Negative capability means being attentive to what will happen and taking responsibility for being receptive to what is needed from you as events unfold. Devotion to your role can help sustain you in negative capability.

FIDELITY

In Chapter 5, fidelity was explored as a virtue of devotion in which you hold something with special regard. It is plausible to describe fidelity as a pillar on which your ethical life is set. Devotion to your patient and to your profession encompasses much of what you do. In terms of ethical assessment, we can promote devotion to the principles of biomedical ethics. In the same way, we can promote devotion to acting for the best outcomes for patients. On the administrative and strategic levels, fidelity can be described as a matter of properly orienting your ethical focus. Know what's important and know your role. This circles back to your oath.

Your oath can be seen as your part of a tacit contract with a patient. The patient's part of the contract is honored as the patient becomes involved in medical care. You don't have a particular patient in front of you when you swear your oath. At the time of your oath, you are taking a global contract with all potential patients that may come under your care. Your oath, then, is your promise to tend to your patients with compassionate care that is given with respect to administrative direction, to strategically work for the best outcomes for your patients.

Fidelity can be explored through the imagery of a contract or a promise. Signing contracts is a form of making a promise. An obligation is taken on through the making of a pledge to behave toward someone in a particular way. To have moral worth, the pledge must be ethically legitimate. That is, there must be ethically defensible reasons for making this pledge. Second, a pledge has moral worth if the agent who makes a legitimate pledge acts with devotion toward the expectations set by the pledge.

Patient expectations are lateral. The contractual expectations your patient has for you in your role are laterally similar to the expectations that your patient has for other nurses and allied health professionals in this healthcare team. The way the patient looks to you to provide care and safety are the same ways that the patient looks to the licensed professional who stands beside you.

When you take your oath, you are taking the same oath as other members of your professional organization. You are taking an oath that is similar to that of other allied health professionals—all orient toward care for patients. The pledges you take in your oaths align you with each other. You are all pointed toward the patient who has comparable expectations for each of you.

Devotion to care for patients necessarily raises the inference that you work in collaboration with other members of the healthcare team. This falls under the scope of your professional practice. With professional integrity, you are acting with devotion alongside your coworkers.

EXERCISE

You've been thinking about what it means to be compassionate to patients. What does it mean to be compassionate toward coworkers? How do these compare?

This alignment doesn't have to be—and won't be—a utopian environment in which close friendships bind everyone in your workplace. In Chapter 3, it was noted that it is possible to act compassionately even toward those for whom you feel no empathy. This is possible when you adopt the willingness to see the person and set aside your own bias. It is also possible when you forgive. In the same way, it is possible to work compassionately alongside your coworkers. Have the willingness to set aside your bias and see your patient. Remember who your oath is for. With this devotion to your patient, you can act with compassionate devotion to your coworkers.

HANDOFF AND DELEGATION

It's not one patient, one nurse. Handoff is a collection of everything everybody has communicated about the patient. It's an all-encompassing communication of patient-specific information. Each nurse and allied health professional can respond to what the patient has presented.

Handoff is standardized for safety. Some events in healthcare are unpredictable. If you can count on that which is predictable while holding to negative capability, you can concentrate on the care you give to your patient. The predictability of a format of communication about a patient who comes into your care helps to place you in the position to be responsive to any developments or sudden changes that might arise in the patient's condition (Cowan, Brunero, Luo, Bilton, & Lamont, 2018).

Handoff is essential to supporting patient care. It provides a foothold for the negative capability you need as you provide interventions during the course of care. To serve as this foothold, you must be able to trust everyone else who has communicated. You accept that veracity has been respected and that all those who have had a hand in this communication have approached it with the proper devotion.

HARMONY

Handoff occurs at transitions where errors might occur. The process of handoff helps to facilitate communication so that healthcare professionals can understand what their role is, and could be, with respect to the patient. Handoff also helps to facilitate a functioning working environment between members of the healthcare team. Harmony is the goal of collaboration.

Plato saw harmony as the social structure of justice. The harmonious society is one in which everyone recognizes their place and performs the work that is appropriate to them. Harmony in society parallels harmony in the individual, where it is virtue. Harmony as virtue is excellence of character in which the different faculties of the soul—appetite, conscience, and rational mind—work in concert, fulfilling their roles as they need to be fulfilled (Plato, 1992). (Think of Plato's image of the horse-drawn chariot, used in Chapter 1.)

In one of his longest books, *The Republic,* Plato opens an exploration of justice by depicting a philosophical conversation between Socrates and several other people. Socrates wants to know what justice is. As he considers the relative merits and demerits of the definitions presented, Socrates comes to uncover a few guiding ideas. First, justice must entail harmony. Second, people of justice should work to benefit themselves by working to benefit others who are in community with them. Among the images Plato uses to illustrate justice is the relationship between a healer and a patient. The healer's commitment to patient demonstrates the kind of harmonious commitment that is essential to justice.

This last point is drawn out as Socrates debates with a particularly energetic debate, a man named Thrasymachus. At one point, Socrates and Thrasymachus discuss what it means to be successful. Thrasymachus insists that being a success means gaining advantage over others. To this point, Thrasymachus has argued that those who are strong should use their influence over those who can't match them in strength. He continues with that theme as he argues that the strong should seek to gain advantage over the weaker. Thrasymachus focuses on competition; on individual gain at the expense of others if necessary. Inherent in this mindset is the assumption that your welfare is not tied to that of other people. The view rests on the assumption that you can succeed while they fail and their failure does not detract from or limit your success.

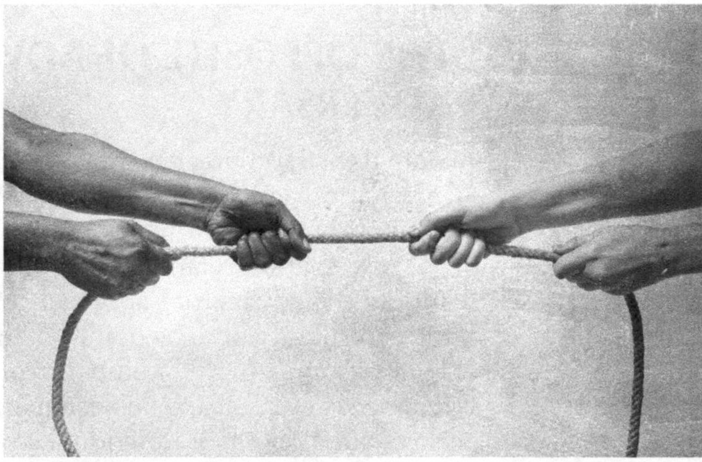

The view Plato portrays through Thrasymachus is an adversarial approach. This view calls upon those who can get away with it to set themselves in opposition to most other people. When alliances are formed, they are formed for the sake of convenience. These alliances are also temporary, to be sacrificed as soon as there is advantage in betraying your allies.

Socrates, the character Plato used to present his argument, works to show that true advantage is not gained over the weaker

Figure 8.2

but on behalf of the weaker. As a health-care professional, for instance, you apply your expertise and art for the benefit of your patient. The advantage you seek to gain is the health outcome of the one who is vulnerable before you—your patient.

EXERCISE

Plato talks about gaining advantage. For now, just think about gaining. What do you want to gain from your profession? What do you want others to gain from your professional work?

In the Platonic mindset, individual success cannot be separated from the wellbeing of one's society. Your efforts to elevate yourself over others have the effect of limiting your possible success just because of the harm done to others—harm that pulls down everyone. As you gain advantage for the weaker, you are also gaining the advantage of your own virtue. This can be reflected in your professional reputation, your developing knowledge and skill base, and in your sense of self-worth.

These attributes of personal virtue also can serve to put you in harmony with others. In the clinical setting, harmony with others is necessary to promote patient outcomes and the culture of safety. In order to promote harmony with others, there needs to be an effort to foster effective collaboration.

THE OPPOSITE OF ADVOCACY: BEING AN ADVERSARY

Plato uses the character Thrasymachus as a foil. He advocates an adversarial approach to social relationships. He views power structures as a competitive arena in which one finds a way to win.

Adversarial relations are based in competition. Someone who adopts the adversarial approach wishes to impose a personal role on the community and, by doing so, pressures other people's roles to shift. This becomes highly competitive. The competitor adopts a mindset that seeks obstacles to be beaten and overcome. The competitive arena plays out as a test of individual strength.

Collaboration is necessary for coordination of care and is essential to patient safety. Introduce competition into this environment and you introduce someone who will create obstacles.

The abuse of professional roles through adversarial behavior places patients at risk. All levels of ethical assessment can invite us to stop there. Needless risk of patient safety is unjustifiable. But further analysis shows that the problem of adversarial behavior can also impact coworkers.

HORIZONTAL AND VERTICAL VIOLENCE

Nurses eat their young.

This statement was introduced by Judith Meissner in 1986. Meissner's article identified behaviors from nurse educators, hospital administrators, and colleagues as practitioners of offenses that amount to an "insidious cannibalism" (Meissner, 1986).

Adversarial encounters between coworkers can be lumped into two categories: vertical violence and horizontal violence. Vertical violence refers to aggressive behavior from someone in a position of authority or seniority to a coworker belonging to a relatively junior station. Horizontal violence describes a circumstance in which the conflict occurs between coworkers in roles of similar status.

Meissner is describing vertical violence involving verbal and nonverbal behaviors. In this type of violence, the source of harm is an abuse of legitimately held authority (Stanley, 2010). This is a violation of fidelity and trust. Inexperienced nurses ought to be able to look to senior nurses for guidance, assistance, support, and for modeling of what a professional nurse should be. Instead, they find a source of grief. The extent of the harm of vertical violence has the potential to lead to cynicism in which the person subject to violence comes to distrust other people in authority and the organization as a whole (Thomas & Burk, 2009).

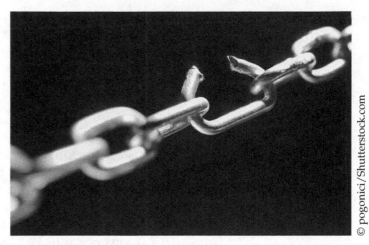

Figure 8.3

© pogonici/Shutterstock.com

EXERCISE

Discuss what it feels like to be in a situation where you are stressed and don't have control. How do you gain control—in healthy or unhealthy ways? What does it feel like to be at the end of someone's effort to exert control?

The aggression of horizontal violence does not involve an abuse of legitimately held power. Even so, it violates fidelity and trust (Stanley, 2010). Fellow health-care professionals share a fundamental pledge to avoid causing harm. For the sake of the professional task and patient outcomes, there has to be trust that coworkers will collaborate. Horizontal violence undermines the expectation other professionals must have for their workplace environment and for their coworkers.

Then there is the harm itself. Depending on the nature of the violence, this can include physical harm. Psychological harm can be inflicted, stemming in part from the violations of trust and fidelity. The experience of harm upends your aspirations for your workplace as well as your expectations for your profession.

At the administrative level, the Kantian perspective of horizontal and vertical violence will be clear. The humanity formulation of the categorical imperative calls upon us to avoid treating people merely as a means to our own ends. Adversarial treatment of a coworker does not show the respect due to a rational being. The coworker is reduced to a mere means to an end. The end—the goal of the violence—itself seems to be doubtful as a rational motive. Why bring about this violence? What good might it serve? Recognizing the importance of collaboration for patient outcomes and safety, a strategic-level assessment will condemn horizontal and vertical violence as well.

EXERCISE

Try a detailed application of the Kantian categorical imperative to the issue of horizontal and vertical violence. Do the principles of biomedical ethics have application here as well?

Note the irony of vertical violence in nursing and allied health. Chapter 5 cited several years of Gallup polls that reveal nursing to be the most trusted professionals. This placement of trust certainly has something to do with a public understanding of the nurse's role as a caregiver. When asked to select the profession that they trust the most, we can imagine members of the public associating caring with trust. And yet, horizontal and vertical violence within nursing and allied health is a recognized issue. Several researchers in addition to Meissner have written about the issue (Meissner, 1999). We might be left with the impression that nurses are adept at caring for patients, but not as much when it comes to caring for other nurses. Thanks to Meissner and to other researchers engaging this issue, we hope that positive directions for change are taking hold (Clarke, Kane, Rajacich, & Lafreniere, 2012). Growing emphasis on collaboration and the culture of safety should also have the effect of working against workplace violence in healthcare.

No one wants to be thought of as uncaring. To be thought of this way is to be discredited in some fashion and subject to stigma. And yet—more irony—those who are targeted for horizontal or vertical violence can be stigmatized by the one committing the violence. Horizontal and vertical violence demonstrate interpersonal bias. Instead of seeing the coworker as a person, the perpetrator of violence sees something else entirely. An obstacle, a threat, a source of more work, a source of stress, a source of jealousy. The adversary sees anything but the person who is hurt by the adversary's behavior.

THE ROLE OF COMPASSION

Horizontal and vertical violence in the workplace are objects of concern. Policies will be in place and there should be procedures outlining mechanisms for reporting concerns and investigative procedures. These measures relate to administrative- and strategic-level thinking. The policies, however, don't create a violence-free environment. This is up to the individuals. This is a matter of individual assessment on all three levels. Be your own legislator and recognize for yourself the need for boundaries around adversarial treatment of coworkers. Think strategically about how you should act. Above all, open yourself to interpersonal regard for your coworkers.

Compassion is not measurable; it is not a strategic objective. It exists on the interpersonal level as a connection between individuals. In compassion, there is a demonstration of trustworthiness, of veracity and fidelity. The compassionate willingness to pay attention to, and be responsive to, someone is the spirit of collaboration. The cultivation of interpersonal skill sets you against an adversarial way of viewing others.

In collaboration, it is important to develop the interpersonal skill of awareness of how other people respond to what you do. We know that our actions are not always received as we intend them. Your intentions are privately yours. No one can see or hear them. They see your actions and hear your words. Knowing your intentions so personally, it is easy for you to assume that other people will respond to your behavior with the intention you have in mind. But this is not always going to be the case. Whether or not it can be said that you bear responsibility for the interpretations of other people, it remains that you are with this other person who bears witness to your behavior. This other person is affected by what you do and what you say. Interpersonally, what you do matters to this person. If you see that this person interprets your behavior as something you did not intend, then this mismatch stands as an interpersonal matter. This should inform your behavior toward this person in the future. It may be the cause now for discussion and an effort to come to an understanding.

TAKEAWAY

Take a moment to review your oath and code of ethics. Review the Ethical Assessment Model at all three levels. Your oath and code point to how you can find good in what you do in the work of health care. Your moral reactions exhibit your potential and instinct for doing good. Your conscientious efforts to add ethical assessment to your practice will hone your ethical skills. Think of how you see yourself as a professional. Think of the care you will give to your patients.

Do you also have aspirations for the kind of professional you will be toward your coworkers? Do you envision yourself working as a member of a team? Do you see yourself as a collaborator? The same ethical skills that will serve your patients can also serve those who work by your side.

CASE STUDIES

CASE STUDY 8.1—TAKING A TURN

Marcell is a nursing assistant. He has recently come on staff after working in a nursing home for five years. Working night shift on an orthopedic floor, Marcell turns his patients every two hours. There is an understanding among staff on the floor that a nurse will be present when patients are repositioned in the first 8 hours after surgery. This way, the repositioning technique can be better controlled, and the nurse can assess for pain, check the surgical site, and auscultate for lung sounds. This is especially important at night so that patients are disturbed as little as possible, helping to promote sleep.

Nurses on the floor have noticed a single-mindedness to Marcell's work. If a nurse is not available when he checks on a patient at the two-hour interval, he will turn the patient himself. Marcell is practiced in doing this task alone from his experience in the nursing home. But it is not part of the promoted culture on this floor. A few nurses have confronted Marcell about this, but he maintains that he knows what he is doing and that he is always mindful of patient safety and comfort.

Use the Ethical Assessment Model to evaluate Marcell's actions. Using this model, how should the team on this orthopedic floor resolve the disagreement?

CASE STUDY 8.2—FROM ED TO PSYCH

Oleta is a 25-year-old female who has been admitted to a medical floor from the Emergency Department. She was brought to the ED after ingesting wood alcohol, believing that it would scour alien listening devices in her digestive tract. Oleta has a past history through this ED and has a diagnosis of paranoid schizoaffective disorder.

Lupe is the nurse who receives Oleta on the medical floor. During her assessment, Lupe realizes that Oleta has wounds on her feet and hasn't eaten all day (or perhaps longer than that). Oleta's hygiene is poor and Lupe would like to address this as well. She finds, too, that she is able to understand Oleta even though the handoff report described her speech as "garbled". Having established communication, Oleta is willing to talk with Lupe and seems to relax in doing so.

Lupe is about to request an order to treat the wounds on Oleta's feet. She is also about to direct a nursing assistant to get shower supplies when the attending physician stops in and reports that he is ordering that Oleta be transferred again. A bed has opened up in the psych unit and he wants to transfer her there immediately. Lupe would like Oleta to remain in the unit for nursing cares. The doctor refuses and maintains the order to move her to psych.

Upon handoff to psych, Lupe reports Oleta's feet wounds and her need for hygiene. The receiving nurse, Vic, nods and looks sympathetic but says that everyone has been put to bed already and the floor is quiet. Oleta's feet and shower will have to wait until tomorrow.

Identify all the points of collaboration in this case. Use the Ethical Assessment Model to evaluate the process of collaboration that follows Oleta from the ED to the psych unit. What, if anything, should have been done differently?

CASE STUDY 8.3—THE DRESSING

Todd is a 59-year-old male who is recovering from a splenectomy. Thalita was Todd's nurse for the 8 am to 8 pm shift. At 8 pm, Thalita hands off Todd's case to So, a nurse who has been with the unit for 3 months. This is her first nursing job. At handoff, Thalita speaks quickly and without pause. So has trouble keeping up as she writes down notes. She asks Thalita to slow down, but Thalita only tells So that she has to keep up. So is intimidated by Thalita's brusqueness and says nothing more.

Later that night, So does an assessment and notices that Todd's bedding needs to be changed. She determines that this is because the wound dressing is saturated. She asks for help from Dijana, a nurse who was hired a month before So. Dijana says, "I had this patient yesterday. I found that I had to change his dressing every four hours as the doctor ordered." So looks up in surprise and says, "I didn't know that his dressing had to be changed every four hours." Dijana is puzzled and asks "Weren't you told that in report?" So says that she wasn't. Or at least she doesn't think so; Thalita went so fast. She doesn't remember Thalita saying anything about changing the dressing, but she wonders if she missed it. Dijana says "Same thing happened to me last night. Thalita reported off to me and didn't say a thing about changing the dressing. I only know about the dressing because I looked in the chart."

Out at the nurse's station, Dijana pulls So aside and says, "We have to see what's going on here. Thalita didn't say a thing. I don't know what it is, but she has something against us."

Use the Ethical Assessment Model to evaluate Thalita's behavior toward So and Dijana. Use the model to explore the options available to So and Dijana. What should they do?

REFERENCES

Clarke, C. M., Kane, D. J., Rajacich, D. L., & Lafreniere, K. D. (2012). Bullying in undergraduate clinical nursing education. *Journal of Nursing Education, 51*(5), 269–276.

Cowan, D., Brunero, S., Luo, X., Bilton, D., & Lamont, S. (2018). Developing a guideline for structured content and process in mental health nursing handover. *International Journal of Mental Health Nursing, 27*(1), 429–439.

Edge, M. S., Fornari, A. B. J., Bittle, C. A., Derelian, D., Kicklighter, J., Pringle, L., . . . , Busey, J. C. (2009). American Dietetic Association/Commission on Dietetic Registration code of ethics for the profession of dietetics and process for consideration of ethics issues. *Journal of the American Dietetic Association, 109*(8), 1461–1467. Retrieved from http://www.eatright-pro.org/~/media/eatrightpro%20files/career/code%20of%20ethics/coe.ashx

McCabe, T. J., & Sambrook, S. (2014). The antecedents, attributes and consequences of trust among nurses and nurse managers: A concept analysis. *International Journal of Nursing Studies, 51*(5), 815–827.

Meissner, J. E. (1986). Nurses: Are we eating our young? *Nursing, 16*(3), 51–53.

Meissner, J. E. (1999). Nurses: Are we still eating our young? *Nursing, 29*(2), 42–44.

Plato, G., (1992). *Republic.* (Grube, M. A., Trans. Revised by Reeve, C. D. C.). Indianapolis: Hackett Publishing Company, Inc.

Stanley, K. M. (2010). Lateral and vertical violence in nursing. *The South Carolina Nurse, XVII,* 10.

Thomas, S. P., & Burk, R. (2009).Junior nursing students' experiences of vertical violence during clinical rotations. *Nursing Outlook, 57*(4), 226–231.

CHAPTER 9

DISASTER ETHICS

OBJECTIVES

After completing this chapter, you will be able to . . .

1. Apply the utilitarian method to the process of reverse triage.

2. Describe compassion and professional oaths as resources in disaster.

3. Utilize death and dying as ways to explore the place of mystery in enduring a disaster and in caring for someone who is subject to a disaster.

4. Parallel and compare the experiences of disaster and disease.

5. Apply the Ethical Assessment Model to chapter exercises and to real-life scenarios.

Box 9.1 End of Life

Among the ethical principles that are fundamental to providing compassionate care at the end of life, the most essential is recognizing that dying is a personal experience and part of the life cycle.

Physician Assistants (PAs) should provide patients with the opportunity to plan for end of life care. Advance directives, living wills, durable power of attorney, and organ donation should be discussed during routine patient visits.

PAs should assure terminally ill patients that their dignity is a priority and that relief of physical and mental suffering is paramount. PAs should exhibit nonjudgmental attitudes and should assure their terminally ill patients that they will not be abandoned. To the extent possible, patient or surrogate preferences should be honored, using the most

(Continued)

appropriate measures consistent with their choices, including alternative and nontraditional treatments. PAs should explain palliative and hospice care and facilitate patient access to those services. End of life care should include assessment and management of psychological, social, and spiritual or religious needs (AAPA, 2013).

INTRODUCTION

Giana Upsdell has been diagnosed with stage IV pancreatic cancer. She has had nonspecific abdominal discomfort for a while but passed it off as what she called an "irritable bowel." Sometimes she worried that she drank too much. She hadn't sought medical attention until recently. Now this. She doesn't have good relationships with family and no close friends. She finds herself alone and is facing eviction because she can no longer work. She feels that she has no resources.

Patients like Giana face catastrophic illness, in which they find their lives devastated. They have little sense of what to do or where to turn. The disaster that happens to one person bears certain parallels to the catastrophe that can happen in, for example, a natural disaster. When disaster happens to one small person, most people in the larger world won't notice. When a disaster impacts thousands, it commands worldwide attention.

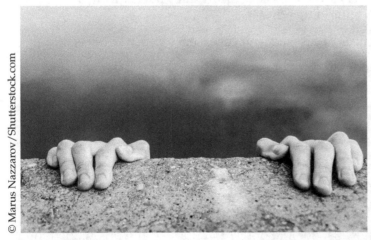

© Marus Nazzarov/Shutterstock.com

Figure 9.1

Disasters small and large present uncertainty and severe threats. The experience of threat incites fear and panic. The threat overlays an even deeper sense of loss. The confusion, the loss of resource, the loss of self, the loss of hope, and the loss of a sense of direction all mean that someone in the midst of disaster can only see disruption. A resolution to the disaster can only be imagined vaguely, just as, in one's normal life, this disaster was unimaginable.

Most of this text is oriented toward your professional life as you operate in what you might regard as your *normal* life. Depending on your role, you might routinely encounter patients who are in the midst of catastrophe. Disasters can happen to one or to a thousand. Disasters for the individual and disasters that are widespread are different in the same way. This chapter aims to address those circumstances, in which everything normal has suddenly been ripped away from your patient. Individual and widespread disasters are the same in that the patient's resources are stripped. In widespread disasters, the resources necessary to treat your patients may be unavailable. Between you and your patient, the same dynamic applies—you are face-to-face with someone in the midst of a disaster.

Patients are aware of a loss of control, whether they experience a traumatic disease or a mass-scale disaster event. The emergence of most disasters cannot be controlled, and they bring a scale of loss and upheaval that can paralyze. Facing an unfamiliar situation, how can a patient know what to do? Facing a loss of resources to act and cope, how can a patient decide?

In the middle of a disaster, it is hard, even impossible, to see an outcome. It can be hard to even think of one. Your focus can be on everything that is happening now. This moment is what you have and this moment demands everything you have to give to it.

What might it even mean to act well in a disaster? Can anyone anticipate what one will do or feel? What can it mean to be at our best when we find ourselves in a situation that we never wanted to be in and that, by its nature, confounds our ability to understand what we are facing? Negative capability is important, keeping you flexible as unpredictable events emerge. Keep in mind the difference between you and your patient. When your patient is in the midst of disaster, you still have the resources of your professional skills.

The upheaval of a disaster means that we cannot know what the experience will be like until it arrives. Part of the trauma of a disaster is that it represents the loss of much of what one understood as a normal and *known* life. The catastrophic life is, then, not one that can be understood before it is experienced. We can study past disasters. We can read memoirs of those who have experienced them. These can help us to build compassion for those who endure disaster and to imagine what it might be like. Imagining never matches reality. Disasters are always new to those who experience them. Reading a memoir from someone who experienced cancer will not let you say, *I know how I will feel because this is what Gilda Radner experienced.* Instead your revelation will be more like, *I had no idea! I thought I knew what Gilda Radner meant, but now that I have my own experience, I see her in a whole new way* (Radner, 2009).

Disaster transforms you epistemically. It provides a new field of experience, complete with perspectives that never could have been known before disaster struck. This transformation of your way of knowing can also lead to personal transformation (Paul, 2014). The new way of seeing the world, and the loss of a world that is familiar and comfortable, can lead to changes in your priorities, focus, sense of identity, and aspirations for the future. Disaster can transform you.

The event of a disaster is different from the experience of a disaster. The event is the environment, in which you have the experience. While the experience cannot be known in advance, preparations can be made for the possibility that the event might occur. Individuals can prepare for the possibility of personal catastrophe by purchasing insurance or by crafting an advance directive. These measures demonstrate some planning in the event that a catastrophe occurs. The person who writes an advance directive cannot know what this experience will be like, but the preparation has value just the same. Similarly, preparations can be made for the event of large-scale disasters. We cannot know what the experience will be like once a disaster occurs—even one that, like a hurricane—we see coming.

Planning for disasters is, of course, highly prudent and a matter of ethical necessity. Strategically, preparation for disasters should enable us to strive for the best outcomes—saving the most lives and as much of needed infrastructure as possible. Administratively, the effort to protect people and provide for their welfare in an emergency can be shown to respect humanity. The principle of beneficence calls upon us to protect people from threats of harm and to rescue them from harm when it occurs despite our best efforts at protection. Ethically, disaster preparation is needed. The nature of disaster means that we need to consider how care needs to alter in times of disaster, and to understand what forms of care need to remain the same (Ozge Karadag & Kerim Hakan, 2012).

ALTERED STANDARDS OF CARE

All disasters are local. This is a common refrain that points to disaster planning. Local preparation is needed in order to ensure that resources are immediately available in the event of a disaster. The use of local resources provides efficiency. Local resources are used first. This provides time to muster resources regionally, nationally, and globally in the event that the local resources become exhausted.

In the interest of public health, we can—and must—undertake preparations to address health-care concerns in the event of a large-scale event. Remember that all disasters are local. To those affected, disaster condenses the patient's world to the sphere of immediate suffering.

Disasters are local in another sense as well. The experience of disaster has the effect of narrowing one's view of the world. As a community struggles to cope with the effects of a tornado, for example, the ability to pay attention to events elsewhere in the world diminishes. You need to keep your focus where the demand is pressing. Within the scope of disaster, full attention must be given to the local.

When a disaster brings uncertainty, the world of the patient and the patient's family can shrink to the bedside. However, in large-scale disasters, the responders and health-care professionals will have many patients with pressing needs.

Standards of care are outcome based. In a disaster, expectations alter. The expectations of patients stay the same, but staff expectations have to change. Standards remain, but they have to alter based on resources and demand. As standards of care alter in the event of a disaster, what happens to the way we approach ethics? What, if anything, has to change about the way we engage ethical assessments? What stays the same?

Disaster preparedness occurs at the administrative level. Policies are put in place to set priorities. Ethically, the principle of justice needs to be respected at the forefront. Large-scale disasters place everyone at risk. Justice insists that everyone must be regarded as equally valuable. This raises the imperative that planning for various disasters must be done with efforts to minimize risks for all populations.

In terms of ethical assessment, disasters especially bring their challenge to the strategic level. Administrative concerns for rights are without context. That is, they remain the same no matter the situation in which we apply them. Beauchamp and Childress' principles may come into conflict depending on the situation, but the conflict is best understood as a strategic choice. In this conflict, we ask, *Which is more important to use as a guide in this case?* The principles still hold administratively. It's in the strategic application of them that we have to make the choice (Al Thobaity, Plummer, & Williams, 2017; Ozge Karadag & Kerim Hakan, 2012).

Such is the case with a large-scale disaster. Here, strategic concerns for how we respect autonomy can give way to strategic concerns for justice and beneficence. Typically, in respecting autonomy, we orient toward a patient who faces a decision that primarily concerns that patient. However, in a large-scale disaster, there are many people who are suffering or at present risk of suffering. Resources are limited, and coordination of those resources is demanding. The interests of many can mean that the self-determination of one doesn't take the same priority as it would under normal circumstances.

Collaboration is just as important in a disaster as in normal circumstances. However, the circumstances in the disaster, such as electricity outages or internet downtime, bring challenges to the collaborative effort. Where the opportunity to communicate has been compromised, veracity and trust are heightened when that communication is present. Chain of command also becomes important for the coordination of care on a larger scale. Veracity from leadership is crucial to establish direction and to reinforce trust.

EXERCISE

Investigate the response to a large-scale disaster. Evaluate the response administratively in terms of Kantian ethics and the principles autonomy, nonmaleficence, beneficence, and justice. What insight does your evaluation provide about how well the response worked? Does your analysis lead you to recommend any different approaches in preparation for future events?

Disasters place us in the position of facing a stark disparity between the way things are and the way we think things ought to be. At its heart, ethics confronts such a difference. Recognizing that things are not quite the way they ought to be—recognizing that we can do better—motivates us to explore how we can improve. Disaster places special demands, dictating the direction we need to go. We can dream ethically about the people we wish to be and the world we wish to bring about. Disaster places limits on the outcomes that might be possible. The strategic task is to make it through, saving as many as we can along the way.

We can feel despair as we realize that we cannot bring about the resolution that we wish to see. It might be that this despair overwhelms. If we cannot fix the whole of the problem, what can be done at all? The worth of a strategic approach can be especially useful as it directs us to assess the circumstances we encounter and to determine what outcomes are possible. In a utilitarian approach, for instance, we assess possible outcomes in light of the resources available to us and the consequences we might bring about. The goal is to seek the best results, not the ideal ones. Despair needs to be regarded as part of an assessment of possibilities. It shows us what cannot be, freeing us to search for what can be.

Under utilitarianism, your decision making remains constant: you seek actions that stand to bring about the best consequences for those involved. Triage engages utilitarian thinking. The aim of triage is to identify the resources you have available and strategize your use of them to bring about the best possible outcomes. Outside of a disaster, in circumstances in which resources are relatively unlimited, critical cases will be treated first. Those who can wait for care will be treated as resources can be spared. In this way, the greatest number of people who need care will receive it in the measure that they need it.

Imagine a scenario in which the food in your refrigerator is all you will have to eat for a month. This food has to last you, your small child, your grandmother, and your adult cousin who is an athlete. If food were plenty and you had assurance that you could readily replenish the supply, the athlete might eat first, because the caloric needs are greater. But now, when you know that this food is all you have, the priorities invert. Your child will eat first and your grandmother second. The athlete will eat last. The athlete will still be hungry, but the athlete will be fed. Everyone eats in this allocation. Everyone might not have as much as they want, but you have made sure that everyone has eaten.

In a disaster in which resources are severely limited with respect to the demands of patient needs, the allocation of resources reverses. In reverse triage, the least critical cases are identified and treated first in order to accommodate the critical cases. The utilitarian goal remains to bring about the greatest net benefit for everyone impacted by the disaster. When resources are severely limited, the allocation of hard resources (medical supplies, bed space, and medications) become a priority. Those whose needs demand the most resources and present the greatest acuity will be taken care of when—if—more of the hard resources can be assigned to them. Sadly, there might not be enough of the hard resources to allocate for all who need them. However, humans are resources, too. Patients who must wait for care are not to be abandoned.

EXERCISE

Discuss the way that a catastrophic illness can necessitate changes in lifestyle, perspective, and priorities for the ill and their family caregivers.

The utilitarian perspective still insists on treating all people with equal respect. Strategies aren't shaped by calculating values for the individuals affected. To properly use utilitarian thinking, strategies have to be shaped by the consequences that accrue among all of these individuals collectively. The aim is to bring about the best possible accrual of consequences. No person is to be regarded as any less than others. If it is possible to benefit all people, then we ought to do so. When demand for health care dramatically outstrips available resources to meet demand, then goals of saving everyone have to give way to more immediate goals of saving as many people as we can.

EXERCISE

Evaluate reverse triage from a utilitarian and from a Kantian perspective. Are these two theoretical approaches in conflict here?

It is sometimes said that, in utilitarianism, the end justifies the means. That is, if the best possible outcome is reached, then whatever means (actions) take us to that outcome are justified. As we see here, ends and means are interdependent. The best possible end that we can seek will depend on the means available. The end we most wish to bring about might not be possible because the means adequate to bringing it about are not available to us.

Because we are aware of this and we are planning, we can direct ourselves to anticipate how we can keep this from happening. How we can arrange our hospital so that we can accommodate more people given the space that we have?

You still provide care. Don't abandon patients. You can always provide some kind of care. Even if compassion is all you have to offer.

In reverse triage, compassion becomes greater as resources become fewer. Compassion and your oath are inexhaustible resources. In tragic circumstances, compassion affirms the person. Kant's categorical imperative applies to the affirmation of humanity—that which makes it possible to categorize all people within the same boundary of morally worthwhile beings. Compassion affirms the individual person. Compassionate attention is to be given to this person as *this person,* not as an instance of a larger group. *This person* suffers. Compassion moves us to see that it is right and fitting that there be at least one witness to who this person is and what this person has lost.

Functioning in disasters, your resources become limited. The first step is to assess what resources you have. No matter what, you still have the true resources of a nurse: your oath, your compassion, and your advocacy for the patient. Just because your resources aren't there, you still are. You still have the ability to care for your patient.

GOOD SAMARITAN

In the United States, all states have Good Samaritan laws. These laws provide some protection from liability for those who stop to offer assistance to people who are in danger or are injured.

The name "Good Samaritan" is taken from a parable in Christian scripture. In this passage, Jesus affirms the commandment "Love your neighbor as yourself" and proceeds to challenge the way that people might commonly draw boundaries around who one's neighbor is. The story tells of a traveling man who is robbed, beaten, and left for dead on the side of a road. A priest comes along. We could assume that the priest might have reason to see this man as his neighbor, but he continues on his way without offering help. Another man, from the beaten man's own tribe, comes along but also continues on his way without offering help. Later, a Samaritan comes by. The Samaritans are of a different and rival tribe. However, this man looks past the differences between the tribes, and sees the wounded person. The Samaritan takes the beaten man to safety and pays for his care.

The story is powerful in many ways. Ethically, the Samaritan's goodness is striking because there are few reasons why he should help the beaten man. There is no expectation of reward. The Samaritan gives of his time, his money, and his physical effort. He gives on behalf of someone who is of a different tribe. He has no reason to expect to see this man again. The two are entirely anonymous to each other, except for this moment of care. All that unites these two men is the need of one and the ability of the other to respond.

EXERCISE

Evaluate a Good Samaritan action from a utilitarian and from a Kantian perspective. Can you envision any circumstance, in which the utilitarian will advise you not to come to the aid of someone who needs your care? Is it possible that these two approaches could come into conflict? How will you use the Ethical Assessment Model in the face of such a conflict?

This is the essence of the interpersonal level of care. The moment of care unites us. Compassion is the willingness to recognize someone as a person worthy of your caring attention—as a neighbor.

BEING WITH THE DYING

In his *Letter to Menoeceus,* Epicurus advised his friend not to fear death. Death is absolutely mysterious. We have already argued that we cannot know what the experience of a disaster will be like until we find ourselves in one. Epicurus makes a similar claim about death. We have no evidence. This complete state of unknowing means that *death is nothing to us*. In other words, there is no point being anxious about death because we simply cannot anticipate what it will be like. We really don't know that there's any reason to be afraid of death.

EXERCISE

Do you fear death? Consider your own emotions surrounding death. How do you feel about facing death in your professional life? What do you see as the ethical aspects of death and dying?

However, death is something to the person who is dying. It is something to those who love the person who is dying. Epicurus' stance is built on seeing the possibility that death is followed by pain or pleasure as unknowable to us. Because we cannot know what it is like, we cannot justify any firm belief about whether death is good—and something to be desired—or bad—and something to be feared. He can help us to recognize that dying is not always bad. Some people find it to be a release. Some find nobility or beauty in death.

Still, in his argument, Epicurus asserts that death is not to be regarded as momentous. The suggestion is that death, or anything else, is only momentous if it presents a significant promise of pain or pleasure.

EXERCISE

How will you use the Ethical Assessment Model to approach an issue in which death is involved? What difference does it make if the death is of a patient, a friend, or a coworker? What is the difference if you are with someone who is dying or present when someone is diagnosed with a terminal condition?

Put this in the context of disaster. In the event of a disaster, one's normal life is catastrophically disrupted. There is loss. There is an ending. Because meaning is lost, it is hard to say that a disaster is meaningful, but it can safely be argued that being subject to this disaster is an experience that cannot be ignored. It demands reckoning. No matter how we try to put death in perspective, it is always unique and unprecedented for the one to whom it happens. Death is a moment. In that moment is a world of change, a universe of significance.

It is perhaps easier to say that the death of someone else is nothing to us. As long as we can hold someone's dying as an abstraction, then we can safely take the perspective that Epicurus advances. From this distance, we can entertain the notion that we have no confidence that death entails any suffering, so we should have no fear. However, on the interpersonal level, you participate with your patient as this person faces death.

There are disasters that you will witness that will persist in your memory. They will present you with questions. They will continue to strike you with the starkness of their mystery. They will not resolve. In time, you might be able to grow around the memory of trauma and pain. Moral residue can persist for some time, but this, too, might fade. Even then, the memory of the event can stay, tinged with its mystery. Here, you find the preciousness of life. In this memory, you recall a person whose life had significance that was unique in all the world. If this memory stays with you, then you have a blessing. Each precious life that has been lost can serve as a reminder of the preciousness of each person that you care for now.

As you are with someone who is dying, let the experience be local. Death in every situation is unique to the moment and the person involved. There is no special advice to offer other than to be open to what the experience presents. Be willing to attend to this. You will still offer comfort care, there will still be orders to follow. As you offer the skills of your clinical care, offer your acknowledgment of the person.

TAKEAWAY

This chapter offers the analogy of disaster with disease. For the patient, traumatic disease or injury is experienced as catastrophe. A disease, like a disaster, has no interpersonal regard for those to whom it happens. In the experience of suffering, disease is personal disaster. Suffering is always personal. The delivery of care is always interpersonal. The skills that you need in the event of a large-scale disaster will be the skills that you need in the treatment of a patient with traumatic illness.

Read this chapter again. Where you read "disaster," substitute "disease."

Remember that, for you, the delivery of your care can be dramatically shaped by the circumstances around you. In a wide-spread disaster event, you might find that the resources available to you are severely limited with respect to the number of patients who need your care. Even then, there are two resources that are always available to you. These are your oath and the compassionate skill that you have to offer. No matter the circumstance, no matter the extent of the disaster, this is always needed by your patient.

CASE STUDIES

CASE STUDY 9.1—FOUR HOURS OF OXYGEN

A series of tornadoes devastate a remote small town. Buildings have collapsed, including the nursing home, the local hospital, and the school (grammar school and high school combined). Infrastructure, including electricity and the one major roadway access to the interstate are severely damaged. Widespread debris and rugged terrain make helicopter access difficult. The devastation at the hospital and the current inaccessibility of the town means the available medical supplies are limited to whatever can be scavenged from the hospital and nursing home along with those that are contained on the ambulances, in the school buildings, and private doctor and dentist practices.

Because there is no clear timetable for when relief services can arrive, the town's volunteer fire department and ambulance service are coordinating the emergency efforts with local doctors who are not among the casualties. At the parking lot of a gas station, a command post has been set up for rapid triage of casualties in order to categorize them according to their injuries. Given limited medical supplies and unknown time of arrival for additional aid, leaders direct that care be given according to reverse triage.

Felix, an EMT, and Caprice, a nurse, are volunteering at the triage site. Caprice assists Felix as he triages the wounded into their appropriate categories: green (minor injuries), yellow (injured but care can be delayed), red (requires immediate care), black (deceased). Under more normal circumstances, those designated as red would be given priority treatment, yellow next, and green last. Felix and Caprice move fast through the gathered casualties, looking for consciousness, breathing, and obvious trauma. Since Felix and Caprice have been informed to perform care according to reverse triage, then they know that minor injuries will be treated first.

As they work, two trucks pull up to the parking lot. More casualties have been brought to the site. In one truck, there are two elderly people who have been recovered from the nursing home. In the other truck, there is a young boy—a third grader—who has been recovered from the wreckage at the school. Felix and Caprice assess the three casualties. Caprice recognizes one of the elderly as her 84-year-old grandmother. Her grandmother is awake but has visible signs of trauma including a collapsed lung. Caprice knows that her grandmother has advanced Parkinson's disease. The elderly man is awake and has only minor injuries. However, he is gasping for air and asks for oxygen. He explains that he has COPD and is on full-time oxygen through a nasal canula. Moving quickly, Felix and Caprice assess the boy. He is unconscious and in respiratory distress due to crushing chest injuries. At the site, they only have 4 hours of oxygen left. With available supplies, they can intubate four people for a total of 1 hour each, or one person for 4 hours, or some other combination.

Ordinarily, giving oxygen requires a doctor's order. Under these circumstances, Felix and Caprice have to decide together how to utilize they oxygen supplies that remain at their site. Using the utilitarian approach specific to reverse triage, how should Felix and Caprice use the remaining oxygen? Beyond the decision about oxygen, what kind of interpersonal care can they give?

CASE STUDY 9.2—SUDDEN DIAGNOSIS

Kofi is a 49-year-old male. He has been brought into the Emergency Department with a fractured leg. Kofi jogs daily. He was out for his usual morning run, when he felt what he described as a cramp in his lower left leg. Then he heard a snapping sound and he was on the ground. Kofi reports no known health issues. He has never been hospitalized before.

X-rays are taken of Kofi's leg. After some time, he is then taken for a CT scan. Back in his room in the ED, Kofi is growing impatient and concerned. Lydia is a nurse in the ED and came on shift while Kofi was in radiology getting the CT. Kofi complains to Lydia about the wait. Lydia says that she will investigate and promises to return shortly. Lydia locates the attending trauma physician, who is in consultation with an orthopedist and an oncologist. They are discussing Kofi's case. X-ray revealed tumors in Kofi's fibula and femur. Based on results from the CT scan, the oncologist suspects that Kofi has prostate cancer, which has metastasized to his bones.

Lydia accompanies the trauma doctor to Kofi's room. The doctor delivers the news. After spending some time with Kofi, the doctor leaves to check on other patients. Lydia remains behind with Kofi.

Use the Ethical Assessment Model. What does Lydia need to be mindful of as she spends this time with Kofi?

CASE STUDY 9.3—TOMA'S FAMILY

Hilde is a nursing assistant who works for a hospice agency. She is doing a home visit for Toma, an 85-year-old male with dementia and congestive heart failure. He is end stage and is experiencing Cheyne–Stokes breathing. Hilde is changing the bedding of Toma's

(Continued)

hospital bed, which is located in his living room. Hilde knows that Toma doesn't have long to live. His family knows this as well. Hilde counts eight people gathered in the living room.

A few members of the family are telling Hilde how to handle Toma. She knows that they are only expressing their concern. She answers politely and continues to do her job. Some members of the family are clearly alarmed by the Cheyne–Stokes breathing. They assume that the irregular breathing pattern is an indication of pain. Some want Hilde to give pain medication. Someone realizes that Hilde can't give pain medication and insists that she calls the doctor. The noise in the room gets louder. As Hilde places Toma's head back on the pillow, he makes eye contact with her. She has been doing this job for a while. She has a sense that Toma is agitated, and she believes that, when some people die, they need stillness. There is too much going on around him.

Use the Ethical Assessment Model to explore Hilde's options. What does she need to do in order to advocate for Toma? What should she do for the family?

REFERENCES

AAPA. (2013). *Guidelines for ethical conduct for the PA profession.* Alexandria, VA: American Academy of Physician Assistants. Retrieved from https://www.aapa.org/wp-content/uploads/2017/02/16-EthicalConduct.pdf

Al Thobaity, A., Plummer, V., & Williams, B. (2017). What are the most common domains of the core competencies of disaster nursing? A scoping review. *International Emergency Nursing, 31,* 64–71.

Ozge Karadag, C., & Kerim Hakan, A. (2012). Ethical dilemmas in disaster medicine. *Iranian Red Crescent Medical Journal, 14*(10), 602–612.

Paul, L. A. (2014). *Transformative experience.* Oxford: Oxford University Press.

Radner, G. (2009). *It's always something.* New York: Simon and Schuster.

CHAPTER 10

SOCIAL JUSTICE

OBJECTIVES

After completing this chapter, you will be able to . . .

1. Familiarize yourself with the concepts of fairness and equality and how they pertain to distributive justice.

2. Critique Plato's notion of harmony as the essence of justice.

3. Facilitate discussion about a right to health and public health issues.

4. Debate social issues pertaining to inequity making use of the theory of justice promoted by John Rawls.

5. Characterize the human tendency to stigmatize others and discuss means to address the problem of stigma.

6. Compose a list of issues that are of concern in social justice and correlate them with opportunities for nurses and allied health professionals to become involved in activism.

7. Apply the Ethical Assessment Model to chapter exercises and to real-life scenarios.

KEY TERMS

- Activism
- Distributive justice
- Diversity
- Equality
- Fairness
- Public health
- Retributive justice
- Stigma

> ### Box 10.1
>
> To provide services based on human need, with compassion and respect for human dignity, unrestricted by consideration of nationality, race, creed, color, or status; to not judge the merits of the patient's request for service, nor allow the patient's socioeconomic status to influence our demeanor or the care that we provide (NAEMT, 2013).

INTRODUCTION

Distributive justice describes a social condition in which goods and services within society are allocated in a fair and equitable manner.

As a principle of biomedical ethics, justice refers to distributive justice. The concern of **distributive justice** is for the goods and services that are available within a society. These goods and services can include such things as opportunities for jobs, salaries and pay scales, access to health care, access to education, access to affordable housing etc. The standard is for these goods and services to be available to members of society in a fair and equitable manner. This is an administrative and strategic view of justice.

Justice also points to an ideal outcome in which everyone has opportunity and respect in a condition of harmony and prosperity—a condition in which important rights are respected. As we saw in exploring the culture of safety, a just society will depend in large measure on a mindset. If a just society depends, for instance, on respect for rights then this respect must be evident throughout various aspects of culture. It is important to have a system of laws that protect rights. However, establishing a system of law does not, by itself, establish a culture. There must also be individuals within society who acknowledge the significance of rights, who think critically about what our rights are, and the relation of rights to law and practice. If rights are necessary to justice then many individuals and institutions within a just society will give some effort to guiding the society toward ever-improving understanding and respect for rights.

If people suffer from injustice, they often seek redress through law. This is an administrative-level focus. Issues of social justice pertain to broad categories, so the focus on addressing injustice at the administrative level is appropriate. Administrative level change requires changes in law, policy, or cultural perspective. As evidenced by the history of struggles for human rights, these can be difficult changes to bring about. When the law brings no remedy, people may seek justice in some other way. At the strategic level, people may engage in activism and outreach. At the interpersonal level, people will seek and rely on the compassionate acknowledgment of their personal worth.

Administrative-level approaches to justice will focus on ideals. Rights will set boundaries, describing what must not be done to individuals in a just society and what must be permitted for individuals in

---

EXERCISE

Often, when people think of justice, they first think of criminal justice, courts, lawsuits and punishments. These concepts belong to retributive justice, which is built on the idea that there is moral good to be attained by punishing people for the commission of certain wrongful acts. Consider the difference between distributive justice and *retributive justice*. As we talk about healthcare ethics, why does it make sense to address distributive justice rather than retributive justice?

---

this society. For there to be a culture of justice, there must also be considerable efforts on the strategic level. The design of justice is to meet a need. The vision of justice should respond to practical needs, such as the need for health care. The boundaries drawn at the administrative level establish ideas of rights that help guide strategic level decisions. Ideas of justice aim to facilitate fairness and equity in the pursuit of real human need.

Justice is participatory. Keeping our attention on distributive justice, we can expect that this condition will be of benefit to everyone in a just society. These benefits need not be simply handed out but can be made available through opportunities established by economic, educational, and other social structures. The viability of these structures will also depend on the participation of members of society.

EXERCISE

When you envision a just society, you're going to extrapolate from what your own experience leads you to believe the social world ought to be. When you are inclined to say that something is not just, where do you see the disconnect between what you see and what ought to be?

Visions of a just society are often expressed in terms of other ideals like fairness and equality. Ideals have an elusive quality. We can debate the finer points of how to draw these lines. We can debate what vision we ought to have in mind as we draw these boundaries. The vision we have of these ideals can shift as we adopt different perspectives or seek to apply these ideals to specific issues. For a deeper exploration of justice in nursing and allied health, we begin with a consideration of the ideals of fairness and equality.

FAIRNESS

Fairness is the treatment of people within a group such that everyone is treated comparably with each other and also in a manner appropriate to individual circumstances.

Fairness is a conceptual principle by which we strive to respect the self-interest of all while also setting up limits on the exercise of self-interest that would be to the detriment of others. The classic statement of fairness as applied to liberty, for instance, is to say that each person should enjoy just as much liberty as we can allow everyone else or until one person's liberty would curtail someone else's similar opportunity to exercise liberty.

A strategic-level view of fairness speaks of treatment of all people on a comparable level. It is set against bias. If bias is opposed to fairness and fairness is essential to justice, then we cannot have a just society unless we cultivate the ability to treat each other without bias.

Before we get too comfortable with the opposition between fairness and bias, consider whether bias can ever be good or, at least, not bad. In Chapter 3 it was asserted that empathy produces bias in moral reactions. Recognizing this bias helps to demonstrate the importance to engage in ethical assessment and modulate moral reactions. Even so, must we view this bias as bad? When bias is bad, what can we identify to recognize it as such? If some bias is the product of intuitive reactions, are we at fault for inherent reactions to events that strike us as morally significant?

We also invoke bias as part of our aspirations and expectations for what the world will be. Patients and health-care professionals often comment that illness isn't fair. This is a matter between the individual and the universe. Or, really, between the individual and the individual's sense of what the universe should be like. Illness is not something that fits with the way we see a just and ordered world. We see health as normal.

If the view of illness as unfair belies an element of bias in our expectations for what our lives ought to be, then perhaps bias is revealed in other aspirations that we have for a good life and a good world. Wouldn't this mean that our expectations for fairness and justice themselves reveal a certain bias in how we view our social world?

Our judgments about fairness and, by extension, justice reflect our own values and beliefs. When people internalize, they want to protect themselves and their vision. Fairness is a type of moral reaction. At least, this is how it often plays out when people complain about something as *unfair*. If somebody says, *That's not fair!* are they just venting an opinion? Is the statement an indication that something amiss with the way they perceive? Maybe it's rather like a nonspecific health complaint—an indication that we need to look for some underlying reason for their outburst.

Fairness can also be a type of reasoned judgment. Our beliefs can come from moral reactions. They can also come from careful ethical assessment. Review the Ethical Assessment Model. You'll see that the model engages you in identifying your own feelings and reactions as it also encourages you to identify different perspectives from other people and from the three levels of assessment. You might be able to identify your own bias in this process. But you should also be able to identify and seriously consider alternative perspectives. As you take these into account, you can apply your critical thinking to arrive at a new perspective.

EXERCISE

Think about something at school or work that is seen as unfair. Select something that you think is unfair or that someone else thinks is unfair. Examine this issue using the Ethical Assessment Model. What deeper perspective can you gain by doing so?

In retrospect, it might be that view of fairness should only be described as biased when they result from reactive views or rationalizations. Views that judge fairness according to a perspective that is the product of critical ethical analysis should, perhaps, be described differently.

If you say that something is unfair, you might feel separated from your beliefs. There's a separation between the way things are and your beliefs about the way things should be. You can work to try to change the world to reconcile the way things are to your beliefs. You can work to try change your beliefs to reconcile your view to the way the world is. The appropriateness of either depends on critical thinking about your beliefs. Should you believe this?

Fairness draws comparisons between two or more people with respect to some third condition. Judgments of fairness are often made with respect to merit or need. For instance, we can critique a reward system according to whether the same rewards are given to different people based on similar merit. Such a distribution of reward is likely to be viewed as fair. We also want to see that these rewards are given with consistency over time in order to deem the system of rewards as fair.

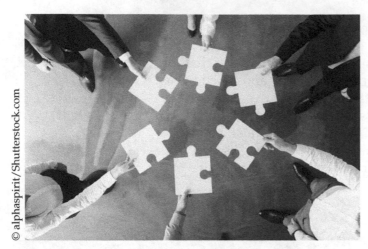

Figure 10.1

Fairness operates at the strategic level. It is the just treatment of people. Just treatment of people involves two main points of focus. First, there is the focus on a group of people. Everyone in that group can be compared in some way such that the treatment of one member of the group is relevant to the way that other members of the group can be treated. Fair treatment here will mean that the treatment of one is deemed reasonable comparable to the treatment of others. The second focus is on an individual within that group. The way this individual is treated might not be precisely the same as the way that other members of the group will be treated. Specific members of the group require treatment that is individualized to their needs. Fairness, then, includes treating people in a manner that is appropriate to them.

Aaliyah is a nurse at a same-day outpatient surgery center. The healthcare system's policies require that tobacco cessation education be offered to each patient on admission. Today, Aaliyah screened a 3-year old male, Wesley; a 16-year old female, Ada; and a 70-year old male, Lonnie. Aaliyah offers tobacco screening to Lonnie. Aaliyah knows that screening for tobacco usage is appropriate in the pediatric setting for teenage patients. She, therefore offers this screening to Ada. She does not offer this screening to Wesley.

Exercise

Discuss Aaliyah's treatment of her three patients. Has she treated the three of them fairly and appropriately?

The just treatment of people is informed by administrative-level assessments of the kind of treatment that ought to be offered to all people based on their categorization as human beings. The concept that applies to this way of drawing boundaries is equality. Equality sets broad standards. Fairness pertains to the application of these standards to individuals within groups, so that each person is treated appropriately for the individual's needs and within the context of the treatment given to everyone in that group.

EQUALITY

Like fairness, **equality** is a comparative concept. Equality compares two or more people with respect to a third element. We can speak of people being equal before the law or possessing equal responsibility for an action.

> **Equality** is a condition in which people in a group are treated similarly with respect to an important point of comparison.

Equality draws its comparison on an administrative level, addressing rights and respect. Equality describes what it means to embrace a spirit of justice as we regard people. In a culture of justice, we hold each person with the same respect we offer to any other person. In a culture of justice, we acknowledge that human rights apply to each and every human being. Notions of equality inform how we treat each other fairly and appropriately.

EXERCISE

Return to Aaliyah's example above. Consider the health-care system's policy that requires that all patients be offered tobacco cessation education upon admission. Discuss how such a policy might respect equality.

Similarity also plays a role in equality. To be equal, we do not insist that people are treated identically. Identical treatment would mean treating one person in the precise manner that another person is treated. It would be inappropriate, for instance, for Aaliyah to treat Wesley identically to the way she treats Ada or Lonnie. Equality entails treating people similarly (the broader focus of fairness), but appropriately. Equality, then, must be a boundary that allows us to acknowledge a group of people for some broad similarity that they share. At the same time, policies that treat these people equally must be broad enough to allow for individualized treatment as appropriate.

When we speak of justice, we think of putting things right. Distributive justice leads us to think about making available goods and services in society in the right measure. When we think of **retributive justice**, we think of correcting wrongs that have been done. In both, we exhibit the tendency to think in terms of treating people according to what they deserve or merit. Desert and merit involve value judgments about the worth of what somebody has done—has earned. In order to return what someone has earned, we look for a reward or a punishment that is of comparable worth to the merit. The idea of giving back to people according to the measure of what they have earned is *reciprocity*.

Retributive justice describes a system within society for responding to wrongdoing such that punishments are doled out according to what offenders deserve.

RECIPROCITY

Reciprocity is built on the idea of like for like. Actions that are done in the past meet with comparable responses in the future. In terms of justice, we can talk about punishments that fit the crime. We often hold the expectation that job offers and pay raises should be given according to what people have earned. When it comes to access to health care, we might argue that all people deserve this as a human right. In other words, humans deserve this access simply on the merit of being human.

We look to reciprocity strategically to guide our responses to what people have done and to the circumstances in which they live. However, strategic judgments based on reciprocity are not at all straightforward. Social debates abound about whether certain crimes deserve punishment or rehabilitation, and about what kind of opportunities ought to be extended to poor and disadvantaged populations. Logistical constraints and policy decisions can present challenges for rewards based on merit. For example, an organization might adopt a budget policy to award raises on a flat percentage rate instead of on an assessment of individual merit.

It is difficult to systematically determine how actions should be repaid in a like-for-like manner. The ancient Code of Hammurabi outlined a list of punishments to be given for certain offenses as a matter of reciprocity. Among the provisions, is a directive that a farmer who, in the process of irrigating his crops accidentally floods his neighbor's fields shall be required to compensate his neighbor for any lost crops. The code also specifies that a thief who steals a pig will be punished differently based on circumstance. If the pig belonged to a temple, the thief would have to pay back 30 pigs. If the thief stole the pig from a friend of the king, the thief would have to pay back 10 pigs. If the thief could not afford to pay the fine, he would be executed (Outman, 2007).

We look to reciprocity as a guide to set things right. Sometimes we find that making things right is a direct matter of restoring what was lost—as in the case of the Code of Hammurabi and the farmer's field. Other times, we judge that restoration is not enough and seek to add greater disincentives to a punishment. Calculating what is sufficient to restore and what is sufficient as added disincentive or incentive is difficult and can be somewhat arbitrary.

A better-known expression of reciprocity is as an ethical guide. This guide is commonly found in all cultures and in all religions. It is simply expressed: *Treat others the way you want to be treated and don't treat them the way you don't want to be treated.* If we take this literally as a strategic guide, then reciprocity is inherently caught in one's own bias. I would treat you on the basis of what I want and value, and this treatment might not align with what you value or need.

EXERCISE

You have a 52-year old female patient, Phyllis, who has just been diagnosed with colorectal cancer. She faces a difficult decision about treatment and has been presented with many options. Phyllis looks at you and asks, "If you were me, what would you do?" How do you respond? Use the Ethical Assessment Model to explore your options.

This is the same concern as raised in the discussion of bias and empathy in Chapter 3. When you respond to someone on the basis of your empathy, you are responding from the mirrored suffering that you feel. You imagine what it would be like to be this person, though with the suffering that you feel. You respond as if you know what it's like to be this other person. But you don't know that. The way you would want to be treated won't let you know precisely how this other person wants to be treated.

EXERCISE

How do you react when someone says to you, "I know exactly how you feel?" Do you believe that this person really knows what your experience is like?

Here, as with the discussion in Chapter 3 and elsewhere, we promote compassion over empathy. Read as a guide for compassion, reciprocity directs us to open ourselves to the suffering and needs of another person. *Treat this person as you would want to be treated*. Think about what this means. Do you want someone to treat you on the basis of what that person would want, or do you want that person to have the willingness to pay attention to your wants and needs?

Reciprocity is that aspect of the interpersonal moment in which one person reaches out for help and another compassionately reaches out to help. The compassionate gesture is an effort to set things right for the one who suffers. This does not always mean that compassion will fix what ails someone or restore that person to health. But compassion helps to positively address the suffering person's feelings of abandonment and isolation. Compassion can reaffirm that this person matters; it can be a demonstration of hope.

In terms of reciprocity, the reward for compassion can be social. As you demonstrate your compassion, others might be inclined to act with compassion and kindness toward you. Compassion, as a pro-social behavior, helps to establish and reinforce strong relationships.

Further, compassion is your willingness to attend to others. Acting with this willingness, you place your focus on the suffering of the person in front of you and not on your own suffering. When you act with empathy, you exhibit the willingness to address the suffering that you feel, and this can bring you more suffering if you continue to observe that other people continue to suffer. When you act compassionately, your willingness is with the other person. In this placement of your attention, you move beyond your own suffering. You avoid that compounding effect of suffering through empathy and you are open to perceiving the reward that might come if the other person responds positively to your compassion.

Compassion is who we are. A reflection of personality. A level of willingness. You can measure the level of your compassion relative to the level of your willingness.

HARMONY

In Chapter 8, some attention was given to Plato's claim that justice is harmony. Plato believed that justice in society parallels virtue in the individual. Both depend on harmony and both impact the other. The more virtuous the people in a society, the more just the social structures will be. The more just the social structures of a society, the more people will be able to cultivate their virtue. Harmony in society is a condition of collaboration in which each person identifies her or his role and commits to performing this role well. Harmony in the individual is a condition in which competing reactions and impulses are modulated by an effort of the rational mind. Plato's view of justice operates on the administrative, strategic, and interpersonal levels.

The view of justice crafted here also holds that all three levels of ethical assessment present a view of justice. Administratively, we describe justice in terms of respect that must be given to all humans. We think of equality as a guide for understanding respect and human rights. Strategically, we demonstrate respect for people as we treat them fairly and appropriately. Interpersonally, justice manifests as we embrace the willingness to treat others with compassion.

Plato's view describes a social ideal. When we talk about social justice, we're usually talking about what changes need to happen and how to bring them about. Justice is forward-looking. Within a culture of justice, people of integrity will give some attention to what needs to change and grow in the society. They will give some effort to the development of needed change.

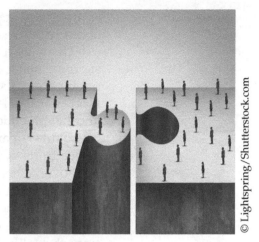

© Lightspring/Shutterstock.com

Figure 10.2

EXERCISE

What needs to change in society? What needs to change in health care? What ideas do you have about how we can move our society forward with respect to the issues you have identified? Explore your ideas using the Ethical Assessment Model.

RIGHT TO HEALTH

A right to health is asserted in the United Nations' *Universal Declaration of Human Rights*. Article 25 states, "Everyone has the right to a standard of living adequate for the health and well-being of himself and of his family, including . . . medical care and necessary social services" (United Nations, 2015). As a statement of rights, this is administrative. It is an affirmation of equality, claiming that everyone deserves the opportunity to the means to pursue wellbeing.

A right to health is asserted as a global, human right. Wherever you travel, you come into contact with people who possess this right. Taking an oath as a health-care professional means, in a way, that your oath and code accompany you wherever you go.

Rights are at the administrative-level of ethical assessment. The right is intended to establish boundaries. From within those boundaries, we are able to explore different ways in which the right can strategically apply. The right to health can be viewed as a way to talk about what we need for a healthy life.

There are a number of essentials to a healthy life. Many of us enjoy such affluence that we think first of access to health care. There are other essentials to a healthy life. People need safe drinking water, safe food that is adequate for nutritional requirements, adequate housing, and health education. Social problems like poverty, homelessness, and inequality all are areas of concern, then, as we look to address a right to health (UNOHCHR & WHO, n.d.).

Poverty, homelessness, inequality, and discrimination all impact the right to health. These impact other rights as well and include health in the scope of their effects. There are other practices that directly impact health. Torture can be argued against as a set of actions that negatively impact health. Nonconsensual medical treatment or experimentation violate patient autonomy and also can be recognized as a violation of a right to health (UNOHCHR & WHO, n.d.).

Violations of a right to health do not necessarily make people ill or injure them. Violations, however, can make people more vulnerable to conditions that can lead them to illness or injury. Violations also make it hard for people to access the care they need to address illness and injury that occur. People are made vulnerable when their right to health is not respected.

EXERCISE

To what extent do violations of a right to health also amount to quieting the voices of vulnerable populations? To what extent do the ill have difficulty being heard? Consider practices that deny mental health services to those in need who belong to underserved populations.

The right to health also describes access that must be available. It is hard to argue that each person has a right to absolutely everything that health care has to offer. The right to health affirms a right to access to at least basic services in health care. This opens a debate as to what constitutes *basic* health services. Strong arguments can be made for maternal and child health services. Arguments can also be made for access to health information and education, and access to needed medications and emergency services (UNOHCHR & WHO, n.d.).

EXERCISE

Define basic health. What must be considered basic health care to which everyone should be have the opportunity to access? What criteria can y ou suggest for how we determine what is, and isn't, basic and essential care? Research different views on this issue.

For all that the right to health covers, it does not imply a right to be healthy. The nature of disease and illness often means, sadly, that health is denied to some. Circumstances that pertain to geography, the supply of medical goods, and the status of medical science all can limit access to health services. Someone who needs an organ transplant is entitled to access to care. This person is not necessarily entitled to an organ.

PUBLIC HEALTH

Many of the needed health services that we infer from a right to health are educational or preventive in nature. These services are in the administrative and strategic interest of *public health*. The roles of nurses and allied health professionals are primarily oriented toward treating disease and injury once they occur, but they are often also in the position to educate patients and the public.

Public health is the science of identifying risks to the health of populations and to identify means of preventing disease and injury.

Public health focuses on prevention. The field of concern here will be more on populations than on the individual who is ill or injured. This large focus is befitting of the primary administrative-level interest in identifying risks and causes of ill-health to communities of people as a whole. Strategic-level decisions will then be made to enact recommendations and policies that extend from these administrative-level efforts. In the interest of prevention, public health is concerned for promoting healthy lifestyle, researching diseases and injury risks, preparing for disasters, identifying populations who are vulnerable to ill-health because of social and economic disparities.

Preventative measures can be offered to the public as a whole in order to prevent occurrences of disease for a few. Perhaps not everyone will be exposed to the measles virus, for instance, but it is recommended that all children receive inoculations in order to secure the health of those few who are so exposed.

A healthy populace is an aspect of a harmonious population. The healthier the people in society, the more they can contribute to the good of all. Due to social and economic disparities, some people in society face greater risks for ill-health. A harmonious society might need to draw particular attention to providing protections for those who are disadvantaged.

EXERCISE

Identify disparities that you see in your own community. How can these disparities impact the health of the people who are disadvantaged because of these disparities? What efforts are being made to address these disparities? Are there other efforts that should be made? Use the Ethical Assessment Model to help build perspective as you answer these questions.

JOHN RAWLS

In *Justice as Fairness* John Rawls outlines a view of a just society. This theory is highlighted by two main principles to guide efforts to promote justice. The first of these states that each person should be granted the same basic liberties that can be granted to all people. This first principle is a fundamental affirmation of rights to autonomy and free choice over the course of one's life (Rawls, 1971).

At this point, Rawls' view of justice is quite similar to a number of other theorists. Rawls then acknowledges that a society in which people enjoy maximum equal liberty operates at its best when the opportunities to exercise those liberties are at a fair and equitable level. If people are so disadvantaged as to find that they do not have important opportunities that other people have, then they suffer. Disadvantage manifests as a basic problem of inequality. If people are so disadvantaged that they do not have the opportunities to exercise their rights to liberty, then they effectively are being denied these rights.

Rawls then puts forward a second principle which holds that some social and economic inequalities are justifiable if those inequalities (a) directly benefit those who are in positions that anyone could conceivably occupy (fair opportunity) and (b) provide the greatest strategic benefit to the disadvantaged and, thereby, to all members of society (difference principle).

For instance, some people live in areas where they do not have access to clean water. This lack of access is a public health issue that places people in these areas at risk for disease and parasitic infection. The disadvantage to this population can mean that many people in these areas will not be able to enjoy the exercise of liberty to which we all have a right. Following the second principle, we can establish social or economic inequalities in order to make sure that everyone has access to clean water. Government could establish regulations to provide for water utilities and require funding that will ensure that clean water is affordable and accessible to all.

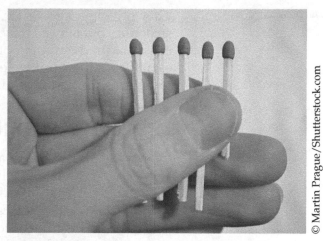

Figure 10.3

EXERCISE

The fair opportunity provision of the second principle states that any inequalities (such as tax incentives, grants, or preferences in obtaining government job contracts) must be made available to positions that anyone could hold. This means that incentives cannot be given directly to people on the basis of factors like chronic illness stemming from genetic conditions, gender, or race. This is a point of some controversy. Discuss this aspect of Rawls' theory. Is the fair opportunity provision genuinely fair?

Looking at both principles from the standpoint of public health provides a perspective that invites us to identify those populations who are at particular risk for disease and injury. The second principle is intended to provide some strategic guidance to address the particular vulnerability of these populations and also the sources of their disadvantage. Also, Rawls' principles invite us to identify those specific risks to public health that stand to devastate and disadvantage populations.

Rawls' principles strive to protect both liberty and equality. The first principle affirms an equal right of everyone to the autonomous exercise of liberty. Social and economic disadvantages can impair the practical exercise of liberty, and therefore create inequalities in society. The second principle is intended as a way to address such inequalities.

This principle allows for inequalities to be brought into the social structure, but only as they promise to correct existing inequalities that cause harm to certain populations within society. The overall aim is to establish administrative-level structures that can be used to guide us to policies that can result in a practical balance of liberty and equality.

DIVERSITY AND JUSTICE

Liberty entails free choice and free expression. It connects with us as we express who we are and what we value. Our backgrounds, cultural influences, and personal histories will vary, making us all different in perspective from each other. Each of us has a unique view on the world and a narrative that cannot be told by anyone else. Enjoying equality does not mean that we are identical. We should be treated as equals, and not with any expectation that we should believe the same things or hold exactly the same values. Respect for equality must also respect diversity. Genuine liberty must embrace the unique attributes that we all bring to our society.

Diversity is the inclusion of multiple perspectives as represented by people with differences in culture, ethnicity, age, gender, sexual orientation, religious affiliation, and other factors.

Diversity lets everyone have their own unique voice and the opportunity to express their true being. Diversity and reconciliation brings us together with respect for our different voices. This reflects the uniqueness of our differences.

A just society isn't going to be a world of people that are exactly what you expect them to be. Somehow the vision of a just society needs to accommodate other people in their diversity. We cannot all relate to each other as we each demand. There are personality differences, differences in needs, differences in experience and perspective. Importantly, we need to recognize differences in power structure, acceptance, and access. There are advantages and disadvantages and there are ways that these can move us apart. How we reconcile all of this is the substance of justice.

EXERCISE

Every community is different. Every community has difference within it. How do you recognize diversity in your own community? How does your community respond to diversity in order to promote harmony and make diversity a strength? Communities can always do better to promote harmony. What can your community do to further make diversity a strength? Use the Ethical Assessment Model to help build your perspective.

On an administrative level, we respect diversity by directing a view toward human rights, not to the rights of preferred groups of humans. Efforts to describe human rights should invite the views of diverse groups, as the experiences of one group are liable to be biased according to the limits of that group's cultural history and perspectives.

Positively, the strategic level will inspire us to invite diverse perspectives as we assess outcomes to be sought. By doing so, we enrich our awareness of what is possible. We can further identify goals that we can share because of, not despite, our differences. Difference should not be seen as something to merely tolerate but as an advantage to our potential for growth.

On the interpersonal level, we are called to see the person. Some people stand out to us as different. We can lapse into a reaction to that difference by seeing that person *as* different. This fuels stereotyping and stigmatization. Be willing to see beyond the difference. That which is different is an aspect of the person. Embrace the difference in order to be open to the person.

STIGMA

A **stigma** is a mark. A stigmatized person has a visible sign. The sign is taken by some as a reason to treat the stigmatized person as somehow less, alien, or threatening. Stigma unfairly renders someone to a reduced or discredited status (Goffman, 1986). It is applied arbitrarily, without sound reason. Stigma is unjust.

Yet stigma happens. That it happens without sound or justifiable reason does not mean that there are no reasons at all when people are stigmatized. We find marks associated with what is unfamiliar or unexpected, with what we don't understand, with what we fear, or with what repels us.

Stigma is a feature about a person that is taken as a reason to discredit that person.

EXERCISE

Why do we stigmatize people? Think about people who are subject to discrimination and oppression. Why are these people stigmatized? What do we miss about these people when we stigmatize them?

Illness can be stigmatized. This can happen to people with chronic and life-threatening illnesses, with mental illness (Corrigan, Morris, Michaels, Rafacz, & Rüsch, 2012; Link, Yang, Phelan, & Collins, 2004; Pope, 2011), with disability, and who suffer from addiction. Those who are ill can belong to groups that are otherwise stigmatized. The elderly, people of different ethnicities, people who don't speak the prevailing language, and people who are prisoners are all examples. Nurses are uniquely positioned to address the social injustice of stigma. In providing compassionate care, you give these patients their respect and dignity—honoring their humanity. As you provide care compassionately, you are combatting stigma.

EXERCISE

How hard is it to manage stigma? If there is information about you that, if publicly known, might discredit you in the eyes of others, what would you have to do in order to manage this information? Consider how stigma relates to privacy concerns.

With compassion, you have to be void of judgment. When we see offense, our emotional response brings us to judge. Compassion is natural, but it requires modulation. And one of the things we modulate against is that kind of judgment—judgment that separates. When we judge, we paint, we label people as other. We categorize them outside of the in-group of normal and acceptable people. We stigmatize.

ACTIVISM AND ADVOCACY

Activism is a concerted campaign to bring about social justice.

Activism, like advocacy, is a call for aid. It might not be a call for aid for oneself but for others. If it is a call for aid for oneself, that call is often shared by others in similar need. Whatever the origin, many of us will hear this call and raise our voices in support.

Yet, how many of us listen to the one who raised the call in the first place? Voices are wasted if they are not given the chance to speak. Voices are wasted if no one pauses long enough to listen. Injustice silences. Stigma stifles a call for aid, substituting a scripted soundtrack in place of the voice of the oppressed.

There are many ways that patients are given a voice. Informed consent, call lights, and health-care professionals who have the willingness to be compassionate toward them all have ways of allowing patients to be heard. Justice operates on all three levels of ethical assessment. All three contribute to our ability to advocate for patients and to help them find voice.

Activism is about building relationships. It is about reconciliation. To bring people back together, there needs to be communication—the call and response of advocacy.

For patient advocacy at the administrative level, policies are crafted to prepare resources for calls for aid. In activism, the administrative level is called to reset boundaries that are presently excluding people unfairly. Calls for policy change will be (should be) evaluated to address social problems.

At the strategic level, decisions are made about treatment to bring about the best outcomes for the one who is suffering. Ideally, these decisions will involve the autonomous participation of the one who is suffering. In activism, the strategic level answers the call for aid to develop and implement plans to affect administrative change. This level also involves plans to deliver needed changes to affected populations.

At the strategic level, collaboration provides a means to advocate for justice. If you perceive a patient or coworker who is being treated unjustly, there are means to report the issue. Give existing channels an opportunity to play their role. Activism means building relationships; so does collaboration.

At the interpersonal level, patient advocacy occurs at the delivery of care. It is compassionate attendance to the patient. Activism, at this level, is compassion to one who is otherwise counted as among an affected population, treating this person *as* this person—as one who is not to be defined on the basis of membership in a stigmatized population. That which stigma denies this person—one's own personhood—is affirmed in compassionate care.

The idea of social justice intimidates some people. The problems seem so large and deep that we doubt our ability to bring about any appreciable change. Or, we want quick and permanent solutions to what is wrong in the world. We want to establish control where we find chaos, and we become frustrated and cynical when we find it difficult to control what we wish we could control.

"Suffering lifts its victim above normal values. While suffering endures there is neither good nor bad, valuable nor invaluable, enemy nor friend. The victim has passed to a region beyond human classification or moral judgments and his suffering is a sufficient claim." Florence Nightingale (Cox, 2010)

TAKEAWAY

The essence of time is change. The present is always in flux. What we find in this moment becomes the past in the next. The past changes as it accrues moments and as the moments are forgotten or altered by memory. The future is an ever-unrealized, always coming to be, a continually shifting, roiling soup of potential. The future changes as the present and past shift.

The phenomenal experience of time takes on many levels. The ethical aspect of time consists of our awareness that we have some power to participate in change. The actions we take now can shift the potential of the future, bringing some outcomes that are realized in some manifestation of the present. We can act based on what we learn from the past. We can act toward a vision we have for the future. Realizing this, we understand ourselves to be agents of change. Realizing that we can make choices about the kinds of changes we can try to bring about and that our choices can have a significant impact on what we, collectively and as individuals, will experience, we further understand that we are moral agents. We can act to change the world, and it matters what we do.

Ethically, there are two main ways to look at how we can be agents for change. The first is the most straightforward: We can act to change circumstances in the world. With every act, we make some difference. When we consciously make decisions about our actions in such a way that are likely to bring about outcomes that have moral value, our decision-making is ethically robust.

The second way to look at change is to realize that our perspectives on the world can change. As we change the way we see, we can gain clarity into the circumstances we face or into the perspectives of other people. As we change—improve—our perspectives, we gain better insight into how we can act to make a positive difference. Improving our perspectives, we can be more effective at bringing about outcomes that have moral value. More, when we improve our perspectives by opening up to the perspectives of others, we can become more compassionate toward them. Not only can we help bring about better outcomes for them, but we also enrich ourselves in the process and connect to others interpersonally, enriching our relationships.

CASE STUDIES

CASE STUDY 10.1—THE FAMILY IN PRE-OP

You are one of three nurses working in the pre-op area at an outpatient surgery center. A patient is brought into pre-op, accompanied by nine family members. Policy at this center is to allow up to two family members to accompany the patient in pre-op. The family is easily identified as part of a reclusive religious group. The family makes no demands, but the space simply isn't available for seven extra people.

As the family crowds into the pre-op area, another nurse says, "Oh no. We can't work like this," and moves to approach the family to confront them with the unit policy. It's clear that this nurse is going to make most of the family members go back out to the waiting area. The third nurse in pre-op steps in front of the other nurse and says, "No, wait!" This nurse approaches the family, gives an introduction and says, "I want you to know that I had a religion class and wrote my term paper about your faith. I understand how important family is to you, and I promise that we will respect your beliefs."

Both of these nurses are focused on administrative-level thinking. One is focused on policy. The other is focused on seeing this family primarily as members of a separate category of people. A strategic decision needs to be made regarding space in pre-op. There also remains interpersonal questions about how to interact with this patient and family, as well as with your coworkers and other patients in pre-op. Use the Ethical Assessment Model to explore the situation and your options. On a larger social scale, what opportunities are there to make a difference regarding issues of diversity and justice?

CASE STUDY 10.2—THE JOB OPPORTUNITY

An outpatient rehabilitation center is hiring a new physical therapist. Under the guidance of the human resources director, the nurse manager has convened a search committee of another nurse, two physical therapists, and two nursing assistants. Out of all the applications received, five candidates have been chosen for interview. All of the candidates are recent graduates from physical therapy programs.

One of the candidates for the position is Sparra. Sparra stood out in the interview process for two reasons. First, she was very personable and knowledgeable in her interview. Second, Sparra is 58-years-old.

Ji is one of the physical therapists on the committee. Ji was very impressed with Sparra's interview and proposes that the committee put Sparra's name forward to be hired. Other members of the committee aren't so sure. All of the concerns focus on Sparra's age. "Physical therapy is a demanding job. How long will her body be able to hold up?" "Will she fit in? She's probably set in her ways." "We don't have paper records. Will she be able to work the computer? Will she be able to learn the technology?"

Use the Ethical Assessment Model to explore how Ji should respond to the way that other members of the committee are treating Sparra's candidacy. On a larger social scale, what opportunities might Ji have to make a difference regarding issues of discrimination?

CASE STUDY 10.3—THE SUBOXONE INCIDENT

Keelan has secured a bed for the night at a homeless shelter. He is a 24-year-old male. He is agitated, rhythmically crosses and uncrosses his arms, clears his throat, marches in place, and mutters to himself. All of this and more are observed by Estelle, a volunteer for the evening at the shelter. Estelle is a nurse at the Emergency Department of the local hospital. She recognizes Keelan's behavior as suggestive of heroin addiction. His behavior is growing more and more frenzied as it seems that he is fighting with himself.

A decision is quickly made as Keelan thrusts a hand into his pocket, extracts a clear plastic sandwich bag and opens it. Keelan pulls a pill out, just as Lynette, another volunteer, arrives and grabs Keelan by the wrist. "You can't take drugs here!" she says. With

(Continued)

difficulty, Keelan informs Lynette that the pill is Suboxone. Estelle observes that Lynette is unimpressed with Suboxone. Though she releases Keelan's wrist, she doesn't release his conscience: "In my mind it's not much different. I suppose you can't help it. I think it's just so unethical to treat your permanent problem with a temporary solution." As Lynette continues, Keelan begins to back away toward the door.

Use the Ethical Assessment Model to evaluate Estelle's options. On a larger social scale, what opportunities might Estelle have to make a difference regarding the kinds of stigma that Keelan experiences?

REFERENCES

Corrigan, P. W., Morris, S. B., Michaels, P. J., Rafacz, J. D., & Rüsch, N. (2012). Challenging the public stigma of mental illness: A meta-analysis of outcome studies. *Psychiatric Services, 63*(10), 963–973.

Cox, M. (2010). *How Florence Nightingale influenced the Red Cross.* London, United Kingdom: The British Red Cross Society. Retrieved from http://blogs.redcross.org.uk/uk/2010/08/how-florence-nightingale-influenced-the-red-cross/

Goffman, E. (1986). Stigma: Notes on the management of spoiled identity. New York: Touchstone..

Link, B. G., Yang, L. H., Phelan, J. C., & Collins, P. Y. (2004). Measuring mental illness stigma. *Schizophrenia Bulletin, 30*(3), 511.

NAEMT. (2013). *Code of ethics and EMT oath.* Clinton, MS: National Association of Emergency Medical Technicians. Retrieved from https://www.naemt.org/about-ems/emt-oath

Outman, R. (2007). *Code of Hammurabi.* Boulder, CO: Lakeside Publishing Group, LLC.

Pope, W. S. (2011). Another face of health care disparity: stigma of mental illness. *Journal of Psychosocial Nursing and Mental Health Services, 49*(9), 27–31.

Rawls, J. (1971). *A theory of justice.* Cambridge, MA: Belknap Press of Harvard University Press.

United Nations. (2015). *Universal declaration of human rights.* Retrieved from http://www.un.org/en/udhrbook/pdf/udhr_booklet_en_web.pdf

UNOHCHR & WHO. (n.d.). The right to health. Geneva, Switzerland: Office of the United Nations High Commissioner for Human Rights and World Health Organization. Retrieved from http://www.ohchr.org/Documents/Publications/Factsheet31.pdf

CHAPTER 11

BIOETHICS, NURSING, AND ALLIED HEALTH

OBJECTIVES

After completing this chapter, you will be able to . . .

1. Summarize the impact of Nazi medical experiments and the Tuskegee Syphilis Study on the development of bioethics.

2. Compare the origins and character of the field of bioethics to the concerns of nursing and allied health professionals.

3. Devise questions and ideas for further inquiry in the field of bioethics, particularly drawing on issues of primary concern to nursing and allied health professionals.

4. Devise questions and ideas for further inquiry in the field of bioethics, particularly drawing on issues of primary concern to patients and their family caregivers.

5. Apply the Ethical Assessment Model to chapter exercises and to real-life scenarios.

KEY TERMS

- Ambiguity
- Belmont Report
- Declaration of Helsinki
- Medical futility
- Nuremberg Code

Box 11.1 Duties to oneself

• Make use of appropriate professional, institutional, or regulatory mechanisms to intervene when witness to abuse or unsafe, incompetent, or unethical practice while supporting colleagues who appropriately notify relevant authorities.

• Promote a culture of research in the radiographic field that will improve the quality of evidence-based recommendations in the future. Confidentiality and informed consent must be evident in research that includes patients and or their records (ISRRT, n.d.).

INTRODUCTION

The medications and devices that we use today are the result of research. The treatments that are available to patients today are due, in part, to people in the past who had been part of research trials. Research today is ongoing so that science and the treatments of disease can continue to advance.

Bioethics is a discipline in which ethics is applied to everything related to health care. It explores care for the sick, public health policy, funding for health care, medical research, marketing of health care, and anything else that applies to the fundamental human experience of taking an interest in one's health. Ethics, too, is of fundamental human interest. In academics, ethics is recognized as a branch of philosophy. Because health and ethics are of such basic concern, many other academic disciplines outside of the health sciences and philosophy take an interest in them.

The broad field of medical humanities is a collective effort by medical professionals, scientists, and members of the humanities. The humanities consist of those disciplines that explore experiences within our lives that are at once felt to be very significant and difficult to study scientifically. Philosophy is one such discipline, as are literature, religion, history, popular culture studies, and the fine and performing arts. Contributions in medical humanities are also made by law, and by social sciences such as sociology, psychology, and anthropology. Bioethics can be seen as a more specific discipline within medical humanities. Many disciplines enter into the field of bioethics.

There has always been an interest in ethics in health care. The field of medicine has an inherent interest in doing good. Despite this interest in doing good—or in some way because of it—the practice and science of medicine has sometimes brought about harm.

It is not the case that the history of health care has always exhibited the concern for addressing and avoiding harm. Sometimes efforts to bring progress in our ability to treat disease run ahead of our moral restraint. Part of the reason is that science has often been held as a *value-neutral enterprise*. This is a claim that a truth-seeking endeavor like science is neither good nor bad in itself. Science needs to be free from biases and sentimentality in order to observe, measure, and discover. Once science makes discoveries, the applications of those discoveries are then subjected to other cultural systems for moral evaluation. This view of science as apart from ethical analysis is questionable. The point here is that many researchers have held something like this attitude that science should not be subject to ethical questions.

In the pursuit of medical advances, experiments have been conducted without first securing patient consent. Some of these experiments have taken place on children and other vulnerable populations.

The history of medical research has also been tainted by the specters of such events as Nazi experiments on prisoners and the Tuskegee Syphilis Study. During World War II, doctors in Germany used prisoners as involuntary test subjects. Experiments ranged from efforts related to the survival of Nazi military personnel, such as pilots shot down over the North Sea. Prisoners were subjected to tests involving low-pressure simulation, rapid descent, and hypothermia. Prisoners were subjected to poisonous gases in order to test antidotes. Prisoners were subjected to bone injuries and bone grafts in order to test new therapies. Prisoners were also exposed to diseases such as tuberculosis and malaria as part of efforts to discover vaccines and therapies. In all cases, there were no efforts to obtain consent and little in the way of efforts to ameliorate suffering. German doctors were also involved in a racially based eugenics program. As part of these efforts, doctors participated in a sterilization program that targeted approximately 3.5 million people belonging to various "undesirable" populations. Cruel experiments were also conducted on prisoners at Auschwitz under the direction of Dr. Josef Mengele.

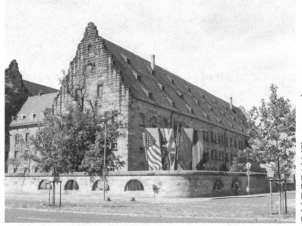

Figure 11.1 The Courthouse in Nuremberg, Germany. Site of the Nuremberg War Crimes Trials

Discovery of the extent of Nazi wartime experiments and the disregard for test subjects came to light during the Nuremberg war crimes trials in 1946. In delivering their judgments against doctors involved in these experiments, judges at Nuremberg accepted six points offered by the prosecution to suggest principles for the ethical treatment of human test subjects. In consultation with medical experts, the judges delivered the 10-point Nuremberg Code.

The **Nuremberg Code** specifies:

- *Voluntary consent must be obtained from human test subjects.*
- *The experiment must yield results that promise real social value and are not simply random observations.*

The **Nuremberg Code** is a set of 10 ethical principles regarding the humane treatment of medical research subjects. It was established in 1947, following revelation of human rights abuses in Nazi medical experimentation.

- *Tests on humans should not be performed until other experiments, such as on animals, have been performed and some assurance of safety to human subjects has been obtained.*
- *The experiment should seek to limit the pain and suffering of human test subjects.*
- *No experiment should be conducted if it is reasonably anticipated to result in death or debilitating injury.*
- *The risk posed to test subjects should not exceed the potential value to be gained by the study.*
- *There must be adequate facilities to treat and protect the subjects against injury or death.*
- *Only qualified persons should conduct research experiments.*
- *The human subject should always have the authority to end participation in the experiment.*
- *The lead researcher must be prepared to end the study at any time that it appears that the experiment will lead to death, injury, or disability* (Nuremberg Code, n.d.).

The Nuremberg Code developed as a judicial ruling. This was the first code that attempted to guide ethical conduct in human research. Although part of the code was crafted because of input from doctors, it was a product of a legal proceeding. The **Declaration of Helsinki** was the first effort from within the medical profession to regulate its own research practices. Building from the principles of the Nuremberg Code, the Declaration of Helsinki brought in more insight from medical research and practice.

The **Declaration of Helsinki** is a set of ethical principles regarding treatment of human research subjects. It was developed in 1964, and first revised in 1975, by the World Medical Association.

The Tuskegee Syphilis Study was conducted in Tuskegee, Alabama, from 1932 to 1972. The study traced the progress of untreated syphilis in African–American men. Test subjects were not informed that they had syphilis. They were told that they had "bad blood." The men were compensated with free meals, medical exams, and funds to offset burial costs. They were denied existing therapies that could treat syphilis, even when penicillin—an effective treatment—became available in 1947 (USPHS, 2017).

The public became aware of the Tuskegee Study in 1972 through a report published by the Associated Press. Public outcry led to the abrupt ending of the trial. The National Research Act (1974) established a commission to develop ethical guidelines for the conduct of research involving human test subjects. A long period of deliberation resulted in the publication of the **Belmont Report:** *Ethical Principles and Guidelines for the Protection of Human Subjects of Research, Report of the National Commission for the Protection of Human Subjects of Biomedical and Behavioral Research* in 1979 (Belmont Report). The report advanced three core principles: respect for persons, beneficence, and justice. These principles are then applied to three areas: informed consent, assessment of risk and benefits, and the selection of human test subjects (National

The **Belmont Report** was published in 1979. It outlined principles and guidelines for the treatment of human subjects in medical research.

Commission for the Protection of Human Subjects of Biomedical and Behavioral Research, 2016).

The first edition of Beauchamp and Childress' *Principles of Biomedical Ethics* was published in 1979. This is the year of the publication of the Belmont Report; the Declaration of Helsinki is still fresh. Bioethics is a new field at this time. There were questions about how to start. What should we rely on for guidance for the ethical practice of health care, for medical research, for public health, and related areas?

Respect for autonomy shows in the Nuremberg Code and is further developed in the Declaration of Helsinki and the Belmont Report. Nonmaleficence, beneficence, and justice also are introduced, discussed, and developed over time. *Principles of Biomedical Ethics* gives systematic examination to these principles, evidencing a developing consensus in the early field of bioethics. It has done so in such a way as to gain widespread acceptance as a forum on which to place ethical discussions about issues in bioethics. While not all bioethicists firmly accept the principles for normative guidance for making decisions in the field, the field generally accepts that these principles are useful as part of the philosophical discussion.

EXERCISE

Discuss the following: Respecting patient autonomy is not the same as treating a patient with compassion. Discuss this in light of involving people as subjects of medical research.

Other medical advances have been less controversial in their research but have brought considerable ethical questions of their own. The capacity to keep patients alive on ventilation led to debates over how we define death and **medical futility**. The ability to grow cell cultures and develop novel treatments from them raises questions about who owns, and should profit from, biological specimens donated by patients.

It is perhaps the stark examples of callous disregard for patient suffering that most attract attention and establish the motivation to specifically apply ethical reasoning to health care. Yet, bioethics isn't driven by concerns about cruelty or wickedness in the practice of medicine. Our ethical systems are already equipped to address outrageous acts of wrongdoing. What drives bioethics is the **ambiguity** presented in the overlap between advances in medical science for the cause of overcoming disease with the fundamental interest to avoid harm. How are we

Medical futility refers to health-care interventions that are not likely to lead to beneficial outcomes for the patient.

Ambiguity is a condition of uncertainty. That which is ambiguous is open to different interpretations, and it is unclear which, if any, interpretation is the right one.

to respond when harm results along with medical progress? When do we see harm as the hard cost of bringing about effective treatment and when do we see the drive for medical progress reach too far?

Bioethics expands ethical consideration outside of the scope of people within a particular profession. Bioethics and nursing offers up the perspective of nurses to the whole of medical ethics and invites others—such as philosophers—in the capacity of their roles and the perspectives and expertise they bring.

Ethics is always changing. It must because people and societies and cultures are always changing. Moreover, medicine is changing—and has changed so much so recently—that there is renewed need to bring ethics to bear on what we do in medicine.

The Nuremberg Code, the Declaration of Helsinki, and the Belmont Report have all focused on the administrative level. Each major step in bioethics has oriented toward developing and promulgating principles. These principles have all addressed significant needs to establish boundaries for the protection of human subjects in research. Strategic-level decisions in the conduct of research and, by extension, in the treatment of patients have been guided by these principles. However, principles only address one aspect of ethical assessment.

As ethics advances, there is worth in expanding its attention to health care by introducing more than an orientation toward principles. It's worth noting that Nuremberg, Helsinki, and Belmont did not include members of the nursing and allied health professions. What is the place of nurses and allied professionals in the future of bioethics? What changes if we bring in bioethics from the administrative level to the interpersonal level of point of care?

Marsha Fowler has argued that the field of bioethics has developed without drawing from the rich historical tradition of nursing. She compares the effort to fit nursing practice into bioethics to trying to wear her father's hand-me-down shirt. It fits, but not all that well. In her reading of the history of nursing ethics, she asserts that the tradition of nursing ethics has always had a "relational motif." The role of nurses places them in relationships with patients, families, other health-care professionals, the profession, and—not to be overlooked—with themselves. The ethical expectation for nurses has traditionally been to respond to these relationships (Fowler, 2017).

Bioethics, meanwhile, has focused more on outlining principles to be followed. This administrative-level orientation draws the field more toward issues that can be examined for broad guidance that can drive strategic decisions. We look to shape boundaries around medical futility, patient autonomy and capacity, brain death, and so on. Efforts into investigating these issues is important, and ongoing research in these areas is needed.

Still, there is room for more efforts to engage the interpersonal roles of nurses and allied health professionals (Saxén, 2018). Respecting a patient's autonomy, while necessary, does not establish a relationship. Providing compassionate care adds an element to the process of obtaining informed consent. This aspect of interacting with patients, families, coworkers, and others is one but one area that nursing and allied health can add to the field of bioethics.

BIOETHICS AND THE PERSPECTIVES OF NURSING AND ALLIED HEALTH

This book offers ethical assessment on three levels: administrative, strategic, and interpersonal. The history of bioethics has so far focused on administrative-level principles and used them to delve into debates over strategic approaches to a number of issues. The chapters in this text outline an approach that strives to bring attention to the interpersonal level along with the administrative and strategic levels of ethical analysis. In doing so, a number of issues are offered that, from a nursing and allied health perspective, might bring new topics and invite new dialogue into the field of bioethics.

Imagine an exercise in which you are to come up with questions for the whole of health care, questions that are generated by nurses and allied health professionals. That's what this chapter is, a series of prompts and an open invitation to bring your thoughts to questions that need to be asked for the good of health care as a whole. Are there matters that pertain to bioethics that are of special concern to nursing and allied health? What do you, in your professional capacity, see that needs to be asked of the health-care community as a whole?

EXERCISE

You encounter a patient, Zephania, who is involved in a research study. Zephania has been describing to you the risks and benefits of the study. You are familiar with this study and you believe that Zephania is overestimating the potential benefits that she might derive as a test subject. You recognize that she has signed an informed consent form and that she has the autonomy to choose to be a participant in the study. How do you interact with Zephania? Ethically, what does Zephania need from you?

Treat the rest of this chapter as an exercise. Read the sections below and think about what you have explored through this book. What further questions, observations, and insights do you have? What directions do you see for further inquiry?

COMPASSION

In this book, the authors have chosen to focus on compassion rather than on care as an ethical skill. This is done with some trepidation, owing to the growing and rich philosophical exploration into caring as a guiding ethical outlook. Much of this literature has taken nursing as a model for ethical behavior, and much of this literature has been embraced—and for good reason—within the field of nursing ethics.

Several reasons stand behind the choice to speak directly to compassion in this book and to treat caring relatively obliquely. First, we wish to avoid potential confusion over caring as an ethical concept and caring as actions directed by a doctor's orders. Although there is clear overlap between these, and doctors' orders must be respected, the two are not identical. A care plan is not an ethics plan.

Second, there is increasing interest in the literature and in related fields to empathy. An observable push is underway to promote empathy as the essence of caring. As noted earlier, empathy is loosely defined and research into empathy raises some concerns about the extent to which we should rely on it for ethical guidance. Compassion is offered as an alternative—one that is not offered as superior to empathy, but as belonging to a different type. Studies of empathy show it to be a component in one's moral reaction. Compassion is presented as a product of critical thinking and ethical assessment.

KINDNESS

Buddhist tradition has informed much of this book's presentation of compassion. Buddhist ethics do not advocate compassion as the sole virtue for ethical guidance. Kindness, or loving-kindness, also has a key role. The authors made a strategic decision not to make this a text that fully embraces Buddhist ethics and found that the flow of the ethical exploration was rather smoother if the interpersonal level of ethics focused on compassion. However, the roles of loving-kindness, along with shared joy and equanimity, are potentially rich areas for ethics in nursing and allied health and in bioethics at large.

MULTILEVELED ETHICAL ASSESSMENT

The Ethical Assessment Model presented throughout the book has application that is not exclusive to nursing and allied health. The model represents an effort to incorporate what are identified as three main perspectives taken in normative ethical theory. The use of this model reveals that the history of bioethics has been strongly oriented toward one of these main perspectives.

The Ethical Assessment Model can be used alongside the patient, even shared with the patient. This can be a way to honor patient autonomy and involve the patient more in the process of understanding and participating in decision-making processes.

The nurse is at the bedside. There, the nurse interfaces with the patient. The patient desires an outcome. The physicians and other members of the health-care team also desire a positive outcome for the patient. Do they all share comparable views of what outcomes ought to be pursued and the reasons for pursuing them? In what ways can the Ethical Assessment Model assist in gathering, comparing, and discussing these views?

PROFESSIONAL INTEGRITY

The pursuit of professional integrity is the pursuit of wholeness in your role as a health-care professional. The ethical attributes of your professional role can extend into your professional life. Your profession becomes a part of who you are personally. Your professional integrity is a key part of your larger pursuit of personal integrity.

Examine the place of your professional oath and code of ethics for your role and for the direction in which you live your life. Your oath is steadfast through your entire career. No matter where you perform your role, no matter what situation you are in, your oath and code are there for you.

Consider the significance with which we treat our professional oaths and codes of ethics in health care. To what extent do we explore what these mean and what they should say? To what extent do we publicly promote these as a declaration of who we are and what we do?

CULTURE OF SAFETY

Bioethics orients toward principles and toward addressing hard strategic decisions to be made in situations where we identify moral conflicts. In addressing health care, bioethics is addressing a culture. In this culture, a mindset that values safety is necessary. The culture is broader and deeper than decisions made for specific situations.

The principle of nonmaleficence is important. Is the respect for this principle sufficient for the development of a culture of safety? What else do we need on the interpersonal and strategic levels to promote and nurture this culture?

ADVOCACY AND VOICE

Advocacy is a call for aid. In what ways are patients' voices heard? Work is being done in the area of narrative ethics. Further exploration into this area with its implications for the interpersonal level of ethical assessment is warranted. Consider all the ways that patients speak. How are their voices heard? What does it mean to advocate for the patient compassionately, rather than relying primarily on empathy?

As we talk about voice, we can also open to the voices of nurses and allied health professionals. What perspectives do they have to offer bioethics that have not been heard?

MORAL DEJECTION

Nursing and allied health are counted among the caring professions. Caring professionals give; they serve. There is no expectation that caring professionals get anything back for the service they deliver. Giving comes with the role.

How much can one give without receiving or being replenished? There is research into phenomena such as compassion fatigue (empathy fatigue), moral distress, and moral residue. Reports of these phenomena point to a need to rethink what we mean about caring professions. How do we sustain nurses emotionally and physically as they start to deplete? Ethically, what can we offer in the care of professionals, too? If our compassion can help to sustain our patients, can it also sustain you and your coworkers?

COLLABORATION

Can bioethics do more to address health care as a cooperative effort? Do we explore the ethics of the continuum of care? Collaboration includes the whole. Is collaboration more than giving orders and reporting? Is there a culture of reciprocity in which collaboration can thrive? Can beneficence toward coworkers, strategic decisions for effective communication, and compassion combine to facilitate this culture?

What problems currently exist in collaboration in health care? Horizontal and vertical violence impact collaboration, professionals, and patient safety. What can bioethics do to recognize and explore the issue, and craft ways to continue to address these problems?

DISASTER ETHICS

To the patient, traumatic illness or injury is experienced as a disaster. To the nurse providing direct care to that patient, the expectations for interpersonal care remain the same. What is it like for the patient who experiences disaster when no one else around the patient shares that perception?

What is it like to provide care in a large-scale disaster? Interpersonal care is still expected. What are the challenges and distractions to giving care in the midst of traumatic circumstances? If the interpersonal level of ethics remains the same, what does change, and how does this impact care?

SOCIAL JUSTICE

What is justice? How can we analyze it from all three levels of ethical assessment? How do we apply it to both society and to the arena of health care? What does it mean to stand for social justice in your professional role? What kind of platform is provided by your participation in your professional organization?

Nursing and allied health work with patients on an individual level. To what extent does the work for justice call upon you to step outside of one-on-one caregiving? Is there a way that direct work with patients amounts to work for justice?

BIOETHICS AND THE PERSPECTIVES OF PATIENTS

Patients also have unique perspectives on health care. Their perspectives also can be brought more into the field of bioethics. Because of their proximity to the bedside, nurses and allied health professionals can have closer insight into some of the concerns of patients. Because advocacy for patients is an expected part of the nurse's professional role, nurses are in position to invite more effort in bioethics to attend to the patient's perspective (Halldorsdottir, 2008).

The patient might not understand disease processes or treatment protocols as well as health-care professionals understand them. However, the patient understands the experience of illness better than the health-care professionals. There is worth in exploring the patient experience on its own merits and not to try to translate patient experience into reports of symptoms.

What happens if we invite patients more directly into bioethics? What do patients say about the need for voice, for example? If our study of patient voice is always given by health-care professionals, are we missing something? Are we open to what patients themselves have to say and understand about illness? Do we see their hopes, expectations, and aspirations? Do we see their hopelessness? If we hear this voice, what impact might it have on bioethics and on the care we provide?

TAKEAWAY

Think about what it means to walk into a patient's room. Most of the time when you come into a patient's presence, you encounter someone who does not want to be there. You often don't meet patients when they are at their best. Patients who are ill or injured do not want to be where they are. They want.

Patients desire. Desire begins with a perception of need. The suffering that comes from illness inspires the desire for restitution back to health. There is nothing that makes us value and desire health more than the experience of its loss. The way we respond to our perception of need can compound our suffering.

When you interact with a patient, you interact with the patient's needs and with the patient's perceptions of need. These will often overlap, but they will rarely be identical. What does it mean to be there for a patient? Is it enough to attend only to the needs as determined by the medical condition? What does it mean to acknowledge the patient as a person, whose interests—and needs—extend beyond the treatment of the disease itself?

As a health-care professional, what are your needs as you fulfill your role? What do you want to do? What do you provide for your patients? Who do you want to be?

Ethics encourages questions even as it strives to present us with ways to look for answers. Ethics, like all of philosophy, asks questions that don't go away (Gadamer, 1996). There is worth in returning to questions relating to your professional integrity. Who should you be in this role? There is worth in returning to questions relating to the care you give. Who is my patient, and what does my patient need from me? Asking these questions is a way to keep yourself oriented toward your oath, toward your code, and toward the care that you give in the moment with your patient. It is a way to show up and be a blessing to someone who needs your care.

Just be willing.

CASE STUDIES

CASE STUDY 11.1—CONSENTING FOR AN EGD

Verna is a very pleasant 78-year-old woman. She has been in the hospital with failure to thrive and chronic nausea. Her doctor has scheduled her to have an upper GI endoscopy (EGD). Verna hasn't been consented yet.

Verna confides to her nurse, Dallas, that she had an EGD when she was in her fifties. She can't remember all the details but she recalls that it didn't go well. She can only say that she had "complications" and that it was a bad experience. Verna doesn't want to upset the doctor, but she is afraid and has questions.

As Dallas is talking with Verna, an orderly arrives to take Verna down for the EGD. The orderly cheerfully asks Verna if she's ready to go. Before Verna can respond, Dallas says, "No. She's not ready to go yet." Dallas calls down to the room where the procedure is to take place. The procedure room nurse answers the phone and Dallas asks if the doctor can come up to Verna's room to consent her and answer her questions. The procedure room nurse says "He's too busy. We've got a packed schedule. Just send her down and we'll consent her here." Dallas suspects that a full consent process is unlikely to happen in the procedure room. They appear to be too rushed. He further suspects that, once in the procedure room, Verna will be too intimidated to ask questions and express her fears.

Dallas continues to hold off the orderly while he calls his nurse manager. The nurse manager doesn't share Dallas' point of view and agrees that a quick consent can be done with Verna in the procedure room. "That's my point," says Dallas. "The consent will be too quick. Consent is supposed to be about the patient, not about getting a form signed."

Use the Ethical Assessment Model to explore Dallas's options. What does he need to do in order to advocate for Verna? Use the Ethical Assessment Model to explore the purpose of the informed consent process from the administrative, strategic, and interpersonal levels.

CASE STUDY 11.2—LOTS

Go back through the book and look through the exercises and case studies. Remember how you answered these before. How have your answers changed now? Think about what the experience of working through this course has brought to you. What do you see differently now?

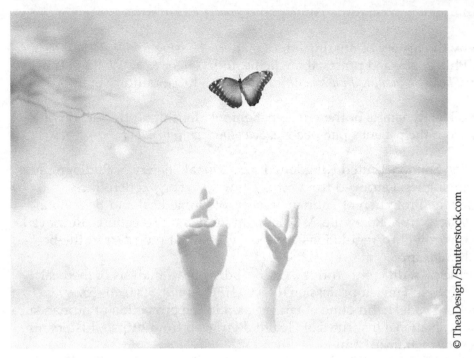

© TheaDesign/Shutterstock.com

Figure 11.2

JUST BE WILLING

Some of the greatest distances we will travel, will not be on our feet but on our knees.

The journey on your feet takes you laterally, in distances measured in miles. The journey on your knees takes you inward . . . into the depths of your being. That cannot be measured.

There, you travel through the soul. You travel through experiences, through worlds that have been, might be and could have been. You travel through YOU. These are wonders that the world cannot match.

Then you return standing, with eyes of greater vision, ears that can hear and a wisdom all too kinder.

REFERENCES

Fowler, M. D. (2017). Why the history of nursing ethics matters. *Nursing Ethics*, 24(3), 292–304.

Gadamer, H.-G. (1996). Philosophy and practical medicine. In J. Gaiger & N. Walker (Trans.). *The enigma of health: The art of healing in a scientific age* (pp. 92–102). Stanford: Stanford University Press.

Halldorsdottir, S. (2008). The dynamics of the nurse–patient relationship: Introduction of a synthesized theory from the patient's perspective. *Scandinavian Journal of Caring Sciences*, 22(4), 643–652.

ISRRT. (n.d.). *Code of ethics*. London, United Kingdom: International Society of Radiographers & Radiological Technologists. Retrieved from https://www.isrrt.org/code-ethics

National Commission for the Protection of Human Subjects of Biomedical and Behavioral Research. (2016). *Belmont Report*. Rockville, MD: Human Research Protections. Retrieved from https://www.hhs.gov/ohrp/regulations-and-policy/belmont-report/read-the-belmont-report/index.html#xapp

Saxén, S. (2018).Same principles, different worlds: A critical discourse analysis of medical ethics and nursing ethics in Finnish professional texts. *HEC Forum*, 30(1), 31–55.

Sparks, J. (2002). Nuremberg code. In timeline of laws related to the protection of human subjects. Office of History: National Institutes of Health. Retrieved from https://history.nih.gov/about/timelines_laws_human.html

U.S. Public Health Service (USPHS). (2017). *The Tuskegee timeline*. Atlanta, GA: CDC. Retrieved from https://www.cdc.gov/tuskegee/timeline.htm

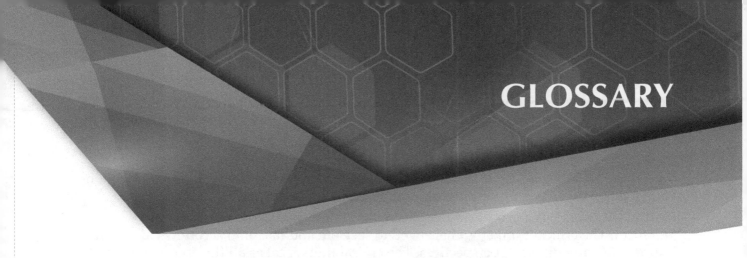

Activism is a concerted campaign to bring about social justice.

Administrative-level ethical assessment focuses on rights and principles that apply to all members of broad category (such as humanity). This level aligns with deontological ethical theories.

An **adversary** is an opponent. Ethically, this is someone who needlessly causes harm or interferes with efforts to grow.

Advocacy is the act of speaking for and supporting someone in need.

Ambiguity is a condition of uncertainty. That which is ambiguous is open to different interpretations, and it is unclear which, if any, interpretation is the right one.

Anticipation describes an attitude in which one prepares for a possible event to occur.

Authentic presence is compassionate attention to another person, affirming the others person's status as someone who matters.

Autonomy is a principle of respect for an individual's right and capacity to make choices that help to determine the course of that individual's life.

The **Belmont Report** was published in 1979. It outlined principles and guidelines for the treatment of human subjects in medical research.

Beneficence is a principle that affirms the importance of doing good.

Blame is an assessment of a moral agent's choice or action, in which fault has been found with that agent's choice or action.

Building perspective is a set of skills in ethical competency entailing the ability to consider different viewpoints with an open and charitable mind.

The **categorical imperative** is Immanuel Kant's test to determine what our moral duties are. It states: "Act always on a maxim that you can will to be a universal law."

Character refers to those qualities and attributes in a human being that marks one's reliability for moral behavior.

A **code of ethics** is a document that outlines the core mission, principles, and virtues of an organization or profession.

Compassion fatigue is a term used to describe a feeling of exhaustion or indifference due to prior excessive feelings of empathy (perhaps better understood as empathy fatigue).

Compassion   is the willingness to be responsive to another person who suffers and to establish an interpersonal connection that affirms the importance and worth of that person.

Confidentiality   is an obligation not to disclose information given without express permission from the source of that information.

Consequentialism   is a style of normative ethics that makes determinations about right or wrong action according to the outcomes produced by those actions.

Critical thinking   is a process of reasoned analysis aimed at arriving at a sound judgment. The critical thinker is challenged to seek out and take into account evidence, new information, and differing perspectives. The critical thinker takes all this information and makes evaluations by making careful inferences.

A **culture of safety**   is an institutional commitment to promote the reduction of risks for harmful events.

Culture   refers to external (language, observances, laws) and internal (values, beliefs, attitudes) elements that are shared by people within a group and, taken together, help give a sense of the identity of people in that group as they belong with each other.

The **Declaration of Helsinki**   is a set of ethical principles regarding treatment of human research subjects. It was developed in 1964, and first revised in 1975, by the World Medical Association.

Deontology   is a normative ethical theory that explores moral duty, typically in the form of principles, rights, and obligations.

Distributive justice   describes a social condition in which goods and services within society are allocated in a fair and equitable manner.

Diversity   is the inclusion of multiple perspectives as represented by people with differences in culture, ethnicity, age, gender, sexual orientation, religious affiliation, and other factors.

Empathy fatigue   is a feeling of exhaustion or indifference due to prior excessive feelings of empathy (more commonly referred to as compassion fatigue).

Empathy   is an experience that follows the observation of pain in another. This experience is characterized by a feeling of pain on the part of the observer that mirrors the pain felt by the other person.

Equality   is a condition in which people in a group are treated similarly with respect to an important point of comparison.

Ethical competency   is proficiency in cultivating and exercising the skills of inquiring into issues of human morality.

An **ethical dilemma**   is a choice of action, the options of which each offer some good. Choosing one option means choosing against some other possible good. An ethical dilemma is symmetrical if the available options promise relatively equal degrees of good. In an asymmetrical dilemma, there is one option that is clearly superior to the others. Still, some good is left unattained by choosing this better option.

Ethical relativism   holds that moral standards and beliefs are shaped by and relative to a number of cultural and personal factors.

Ethics   an activity of critical thinking in which we examine beliefs about morality and the processes by which we come to have our moral beliefs.

Eudaimonia   is the Aristotelian concept of the highest state of virtue.

Executive control   consists of consciously directed cognitive processes that modulate other processes in order to pursue certain goals.

An **expectation**   is a belief that something you should happen.

Fairness   is the treatment of people within a group such that everyone is treated comparably with each other and also in a manner appropriate to individual circumstances.

Fidelity   is devotion to a person or cause, characterized by loyalty and advocacy.

Fiduciary   describes a relationship, such as a professional relationship, that is built on trust.

Forgiveness   is absence of judgment or blame toward one who has been accused of doing wrong.

Gathering facts   is a set of skills in ethical competency entailing the ability to objectively and thoroughly assess a moral situation.

Gratification   is a feeling of pleasure at the satisfaction of a goal.

Guilt   is a feeling of remorse for an act that one believes has violated a moral standard and that one is responsible for that act.

Harm   is damage or offense experienced by a person.

The **humanity formulation of the categorical imperative**   is a reformulated expression of Immanuel Kant's categorical imperative. It states: "Act in such a way that you treat humanity, yourself as well as any other person, never merely as a means to your own ends, but always at the same time as an end."

As a moral quality, **humility** is the recognition that your moral value is not greater than anyone else's and that your moral beliefs might not contain all the answers.

Integrity   is a condition of virtue in which the self is whole, harmonious, and intact.

Interpersonal-level ethical assessment   focuses on establishing strong and healthful relationships among persons. This level aligns with ethics of care and ethics of compassion.

Just culture   is a conceptual model that favors learning lessons rather than punishing people for making errors.

Justice   is a principle requiring fair and equitable distribution of resources, including access to health-care services.

A **maxim**   is a principle of action that connects an action with the reasons to perform it under certain circumstances.

Medical futility   refers to health-care interventions that are not likely to lead to beneficial outcomes for the patient.

A **moral agent**   is a person who can make a decision to act in one's social world and who recognizes some responsibility to make those choices in a way that can be recognized as "right".

Moral conflict   A moral conflict is the perception of an inconsistency between a moral value of your own and either the values of someone else or a situation in which you cannot successfully act to promote your moral value.

Moral dejection   is a general term referring to a feeling of low spirits extending from a realization that one cannot bring about the moral good that one wishes.

Moral distress   describes the condition in which external constraints prevent you from doing the right thing.

Moral residue   is a feeling of regret or guilt the extends from participating in an ethical dilemma.

Morality   consists of beliefs you hold about values as they apply to human behavior.

Moralize   to moralize is to take on an air of authority in professing your opinions about morality. It is to act as if others should regard your moral standards as the standards they ought to accept.

Narrative   refers to an effort by people to identify meaning in their lives. This is done through the telling, and receiving, of a story of who that person is and with whom that person belongs.

Negative capability   is an attitude in which one is able to surrender a need to be fully in control and to be certain about is happening and will happen. It is the capacity to face uncertainty and still function.

Negative rights   pertain to an entitlement that persons have not to be treated in certain ways.

Nonmaleficence   is a principle that affirms our responsibility to avoid causing needless harm to persons.

Normative ethics   is that branch of philosophical ethics that examines questions about how one ought to act and who one ought to be.

Normative   is a term that describes the promotion or determination of a standard, or the evaluation of a standard. Normative ethics consists of efforts to help us determine how we should act.

The **Nuremberg Code**   is a set of 10 ethical principles regarding the humane treatment of medical research subjects. It was established in 1947, following revelation of human rights abuses in Nazi medical experimentation.

An **oath**   is a vow or promise that makes a declaration about one's future behavior and can serve as a guide.

Positive rights   pertain to entitlements that persons have to make certain claims.

A **principle**   is a fundamental proposition that guides action.

Privacy   is an individual's right to determine who has access to certain information about that individual.

Public health   is the science of identifying risks to the health of populations and to identify means of preventing disease and injury.

Rationalize   to rationalize is to attempt to justify one's behavior by offering reasons that sound plausible but really don't hold up to logical scrutiny.

Reciprocity   is a mutual exchange of like for like. It can be thought of as a matter of merit in which good is rewarded with good and bad is punished with bad. Or, it can describe an interpersonal connection in which a caring gesture by one person toward another helps both people mutually.

Retributive justice   describes a system within society for responding to wrongdoing such that punishments are doled out according to what offenders deserve.

A **right**   is a moral entitlement.

A **role model**   is someone who is accepted as a person who presents an example worth imitating in one's own behavior.

Stigma   is a feature about a person that is taken as a reason to discredit that person.

Strategic-level ethical assessment   focuses on bringing about the best outcomes. This level aligns with consequentialist ethical theories, such as utilitarianism.

Suffering   is a quality of personal experience characterized by pain, distress, or other negative perceptions.

Tolerance   is the capacity to endure something that is a source of hardship or distress. Ethically, it pertains to restraint in expressing moral judgment.

Transparency   describes the disclosure of truth, providing clarity about what is known and revealing the lack of any hidden agenda.

Trust   is an expectation that another has the skills of being trustworthy. Trust is having the belief that someone will assume responsibility and meet expectations.

Trustworthiness   is the skill set that demonstrates that one will strive to live up to the expectations of those who place trust and take all care to avoid causing them harm.

Utilitarianism   is a normative ethical theory that advocates a decision-making method that promotes acting to produce the best overall consequences for the greatest number of people.

Veracity   is the responsibility to provide accurate and objective information.

Virtue   is excellence of character, or excellence in character traits.

Vulnerability   is the state of being exposed to harm and to risk of further harm.

Willingness   is an attitude in which one opens to the suffering and personhood of another.

CPSIA information can be obtained
at www.ICGtesting.com
Printed in the USA
LVHW03s2236240718
584841LV00007B/27/P

9 781524 967123